Sex and the Japanese

Other Books by Boyé Lafayette De Mente

Japanese Etiquette and Ethics in Business
Korean Business Etiquette
Korean in Plain English
Japanese in Plain English
Chinese Etiquette & Ethics in Business
Businessman's Quick-Guide to Japan
Japan Made Easy—All You Need to Know
   to Enjoy Japan
Dining in Japan / Shopping in Japan
Etiquette Guide to Japan
Instant Japanese / Survival Japanese
Japan's Cultural Code Words
Chinese in Plain English
China's Cultural Code Words
I Like You, Gringo-But! (with Mario de la Fuente)
Korea's Business & Cultural Code Words
KATA—The Key to Understanding and Dealing with the Japanese
Asian Face Reading
The Japanese Samurai Code:—Classic Strategies for Success
Samurai Strategies—42 Martial Secrets from Musashi's "Book of
   Five Rings"
Instant Chinese / Survival Chinese
Instant Korean / Survival Korean
Which Side of Your Brain Am I Talking To?
The Advantages of Using Both Sides of Your Brain!
Once a Fool—From Japan to Alaska by Amphibious Jeep
Samurai Principles & Practices that Will Help Preteens and Teens
   in School, Sports, Social Activities and Choosing Careers!

Sex and the Japanese

The Sensual Side of Japan

Boyé Lafayette De Mente

TUTTLE PUBLISHING
Tokyo • Rutland, Vermont • Singapore

Published by Tuttle Publishing, an imprint of Periplus Editions (HK) Ltd., with editorial offices at 364 Innovation Drive, North Clarendon, Vermont 05759 and 130 Joo Seng Road, #06-01/03, Singapore 368357.

ISBN: 0-8048-3826-7
ISBN: 978-0-8048-3826-9

Distributed by

North America, Latin America & Europe
Tuttle Publishing,
364 Innovation Drive
North Clarendon, VT 05759-9436
Tel: (802) 773-8930   Fax: (802) 773-6993
Email: info@tuttlepublishing.com
www.tuttlepublishing.com

Japan
Tuttle Publishing,
Yaekari Building, 3rd Floor
5-4-12 Osaki, Shinagawa-ku, Tokyo 141 0032
Tel: (03) 5437-0171   Fax: (03) 5437-0755
Email: tuttle-sales@gol.com

Asia Pacific
Berkeley Books Pte. Ltd.
130 Joo Seng Road, #06-01/03, Singapore 368357
Tel: (65) 6280-1330   Fax: (65) 6280-6290
Email: inquiries@periplus.com.sg
www.periplus.com

Printed in Singapore
10 09 08 07 06   6 5 4 3 2 1

TUTTLE PUBLISHING® is a registered trademark of Tuttle Publishing, a division of Periplus Editions (HK) Ltd.

Contents

PREFACE

The Language of Love

There is a saying in Japan that a man needs three things to be successful with women: aggressiveness—*oshi* (oh-she); money—*okane* (oh-kah-nay) and a good figure—*sugata* (sue-gah-tah).

This saying originally applied to the "Floating World" of the geisha, cabaret hostesses, and other "women of the night." It is still true today but in the "New Japan," which dates from the 1970s, there are other things that are equally important.

There is no similar saying that applies to women, since they are generally seen as the pursuees rather than the pursuers, but there is no mystery about the women in Japan who are the most successful at attracting—and keeping—men.

In addition to a pleasing feminine appearance and feminine behavior that brings men into their net they know how to titillate and tease, massage the male ego, satisfy the male lust, and surreptitiously get men to do what they want them to do.

For both men and women there is a fourth key to a successful love life in Japan—and that is an acceptable attitude, good manners, and being well-dressed.

During the long Tokugawa Shogunate the apparel the Japanese could wear was prescribed by the shogunate, and was based on social class and occupation. This made all Japanese extraordinarily sensitive to style of dress in all of its definitions, and being well-dressed today is often enough to get you through many doors.

Foreign bachelors and bachelorettes in Japan face a number of special cultural challenges that go beyond physical appearance and behavior, but they also benefit significantly— without any effort on their part—from other cultural factors that are an integral part of the Japanese character.

Among the things that should be in the foreign lover's arsenal are an understanding of the background of love in Japan, an appreciation of the finer points of Japan's culture as it relates to human sexuality and male-female relations. Also, some familiarity with the language of love adds to success in a technical sense as well as to the ambience and charm of love Japanese style.

While a growing number of young Japanese—especially women—are able to communicate in English fairly well, the foreign lover in Japan who cannot speak at least some Japanese is seriously handicapped.

Learning enough Japanese to communicate on a basic level is not as difficult as it first appears. The language is based on combinations of only six key sounds. These six sounds are the basis of an "alphabet" of some 100 syllables that make up all of the words in the language. The pronunciation of these syllables is very similar to that of Spanish and Latin.

I have included a chart of all of the syllables in the Japanese language, along with a euphonic pronunciation guide for each syllable. By following the very simple guides you can teach yourself to pronounce Japanese properly in the next half hour. Thereafter, learning enough Japanese to become a more effective lover is a relatively simple matter.

In fact, much of the charm and pleasure of learning how to love in Japan is the communication process—the spoken as well as the non-verbal language. The reason for this is quite simple. The culture of Japan is bound up in key words in the language.

These key words serve as doorways to understanding the attitudes and behavior of the Japanese and how to communicate with them clearly and effectively.

Boyé Lafayette De Mente
Tokyo, Japan

Japanese Pronunciation Guide

As noted above, the Japanese language is very easy to pronounce. It is made up of precise syllables that are based on just five vowel sounds: *a* (ah), *i* (ee), *u* (oo as in boo), *e* (as in eh), and *o* (as in so). When consonant sounds are added to these vowel sounds, syllables are created which follow the same sound pattern: *ka* (kah), *ki* (kee), *ku* (koo), *ke* (kay), *ko* (koe); *sa* (sah), *shi* (she), *su* (sue), *se* (say), *so* (soe), and so forth.

All you have to do to pronounce these syllables (and the words they make up) correctly, is to voice them according to the phonetics shown in the chart below. When you pronounce the Japanese words and phrases phonetically, the sounds come out "in Japanese."

Here are all of the syllables that make up the sounds in the Japanese language, along with their approximate phonetic equivalents.

PRONOUNCIATION CHART

A	I	U	E	O		YA	YU	YO	
ah	ee	oo	eh	oh		Yah	yoo	yoe	

KA	KI	KU	KE	KO		RA	RI	RU	RE	RO
kah	kee	koo	kay	koe		Rah	ree	rue	ray	roe

SA	SHI	SU	SE	SO		GA	GI	GU	GE	GO
sah	she	sue	say	so		Gah	ghee	goo	gay	go

TA	CHI	TSU	TE	TO		ZA	ZI	ZU	ZE	ZO
tah	chee	t'sue	tay	toe		Zah	jee	zoo	zay	zoe

NA	NI	NU	NE	NO		DA	JI	ZU	DE	DO
nah	nee	noo	nay	no		Dah	jee	zoo	day	doe

HA	HI	FU	HE	HO		BA	BI	BU	BE	BO
hah	hee	who	hay	hoe		Bah	bee	boo	bay	boe

MA	MI	MU	ME	MO		PA	PI	PU	PE	PO
mah	mee	moo	may	moe		Pah	pee	poo	pay	poe

The R sound in Japanese is close to the L sound in English, requiring a slight trilling to get it right. It resembles the R sound in Spanish. Note that the D and Z sounds are the same in the pronunciations of Zi and Ji.

The following syllables are combinations of some of those appearing above, with two primary syllables combined into one simply by merging the pronunciations.

RYA	RYU	RYO
r'yah	r'yoo	r'yoe (Roll the R a bit)

Pronounced in "slow motion" these syllables can be represented as ree-yah; ree-yuu and ree-yoh.

MYA	MYU	MYO
m'yah	m'yoo	m'yoe

Similarly, these syllables can be read as mee-yah; me-yuu and me-yoh, and so on down the list. Keep in mind, however, that all of these combined two-in-one syllables sounds should be pronounced as one syllable, not two.

NYA	NYU	NYO	PYA	PYU	PYO
n'yah	n'yoo	n'yoe	p'yah	p'yoo	p'yoe

HYA	HYU	HYO	BYA	BYU	BYO
h'yah	h'yoo	h'yoe	b'yah	b'yoo	b'yoe

CHA	CHU	CHO	JA	JU	JO
Chah	choo	choe	jah	joo	joe

SHA	SHU	SHO	GYA	GYU	GYO
shah	shoo	show	g'yah	g'yoo	g'yoe

KYA	KYU	KYO	
k'yah	cue	k'yoe	N (en) (as the "n" in the word bond)

In Japanese, the H and G sounds are always pronounced "hard" as in "how" and "go". There are no true L or V sounds in Japanese; thus they do not appear in the list of syllables. When the Japanese attempt to pronounce these sounds in English words, the L comes out as R and the V comes out as B.

There are long, short, and silent vowels in Japanese, as well as double consonants. But you do not have to be overly concerned about long vowels or double consonants when using this book, because the correct pronunciation is generally accounted for in the phonetics.

To get the most out of this guide, first practice pronouncing the syllables—out loud—until you can enunciate each one easily without having to think about it. Before long you will be able to recognize individual syllables in the Japanese words you hear.

Then go to the key-word and key-phrase portion of the book and practice pronouncing the phonetics for each word and sentence, repeating the words and sentences aloud until you can get them out in a smooth flow.

CHAPTER 1

Sex without Sin

The Judeo-Christian concept of recreational sex as sinful and abhorrent in the eyes of an all-powerful god is, I believe, one of the biggest con-jobs ever foisted on any group of mankind. The ulterior motive of the creators of this concept was, of course, political and social control (especially of women), and had nothing whatsoever to do with morality or saving "immortal souls."

To make the system work, the creators of this concept had to separate the human body into two parts, the physical and the spiritual. The body, according to the Church, was of the earth, inherently vile and sinful, not to be trusted, and not to be satisfied because its sensual needs were the work of the Devil.

The spirit or soul, on the other hand, was of heaven and

divine, and the only way it could be kept pure was to deny the body physical pleasures, especially those having to do with sex.

This view of human sexuality, which derived from the gonadal obsession of ancient tribal leaders to exercise total chauvinistic, political and social power over tribal members, created a legacy that consigned their cultural descendants to a sexual purgatory in which life was one long nightmare of imaginary sin.

Throughout their history, Jewish, Christian and Islamic religious have obsessively dwelt on the theme that human sexuality is another word for sin and evil, and that women, because they are more sexual than men, must be repressed to keep their sexuality under control.

The men of ancient Japan were wiser than their Western counterparts. The gods they created were far more human, far more tolerant than the Western god. Their gods were conspicuously male and female, single and married, and they engaged in sexual as well as other sensual activities with all the gusto gods can muster.

Of course, Japanese men were not so enlightened as to look upon women as their equals. The world of Japan was until very recently a man's world in which the primary role of women was that of child-bearer, worker, and—when young and attractive—as instrument of pleasure. But the Japanese recognized and accepted the basic fact that the body, mind, and soul cannot be treated separately, that what affects one affects all.

The social system fashioned by the Japanese was based on their observations of real life, of nature in all of its diversity, rather than on an abstract theology that treated men—and especially women—as puppets on strings, born with an overload of crushing guilt.

But it was not until recent decades that Japanese women as well as men became free to take advantage of this enlightened attitude toward sex—and the United States was to play a vital role in this fundamental change in male-female relations in Japan.

CHAPTER 2

Heritage of the Fertility Cult

The first Japanese saw that all animate life was created by the sexual union of the male and female. They incorporated this reality into their indigenous religion, which eventually came to be known as *Shinto*, or "The Way of the Gods."

The core of Shintoism is the relationship that exists between tangible life and the unseen forces that affect and control nature, usually represented by gods. The practice of Shintoism is aimed at maintaining a harmonious relationship between life and the gods.

Since constant re-creation is essential to have an ongoing world, fertility—the ability to reproduce—was therefore the heart of Shintoism. In simplistic terms, Shintoism was sex worship, cloaked, of course, in the guise of crop festivals and ancestor worship.

On the human side, one of the most conspicuous symbols of fertility is the erect male organ. Until very recent decades there were hundreds of thousands of replicas of the male organ, carved in stone or wood, lining the roadways and byways of Japan as daily reminders of the importance of sexual union in the survival of mankind.

Some of these penile carvings were huge in size, suggesting (to me, at least) that there was a strong element of pleasure as well as humor in the practice of Shintoism.

Until the latter decades of the 20th century these roadside reminders of human sexuality were still fairly common in the countryside, and I had a lot of fun calling attention to them when I was in the company of young women. I will always regret that I didn't make a collection of them to later position around my backyard.

Use of the male organ as both the symbol of human fecundity and as a talisman for women wanting to become pregnant has not died out in Japan. Far from it. There are still a number of Shinto shrines around the country that have annual festivals featuring authentic-looking replicas of male penises as links to the god of fertility.

These festivals consist of huge wooden carvings of the male organ, some of them appropriately colored for authenticity, being carried through the streets on wheeled vehicles to be admired by the crowds that gather for the occasions. Wives wanting to become pregnant may stroke the penises as they pass by. At the shrines sponsoring the festivals, purse-sized replicas of penises are sold by priests to women who want to carry them around in the hope that some of the power of the talisman will rub off on them.

Interestingly enough, men today, and especially foreign men, are more likely than women to be embarrassed by the extraordinary spectacle of a 20-foot-long penis being pulled through the streets while cheering crowds line the sidewalks.

Of course, part of this uneasiness may be sheer intimidation, since the impression made by a log-sized long phallus is a pretty hard act to follow.

Be that as it may, the legacy that Shintoism bequeathed to Japan played a central role in the overall sexual attitudes and practices shaping the traditional culture of the country, and set the stage for what an unenlightened Western visitor in the 1600s described as "an orgy of licentious behavior from one end of the country to the other."

CHAPTER 3

The Dao Sex Syndrome

Shintoism was not the only influence on the traditional Japanese attitude toward sex and the various social customs that were to develop during the long shogunate and feudal ages.

Some time after the great Chinese sage Lao Zi formulated the philosophy that was to become known as Daoism, some of the followers of the Way of Daoism developed a new school of Daoistic thought that incorporated a very strong sexual element.

They surmised that in order for human beings, and again especially men, to stay in harmony with the cosmos it was necessary to expel on a daily basis all of the sexual energy that accumulates in the body.

These learned philosophers recognized that failure to engage in sexual activity on a regular basis results in the buildup of a kind of sexual energy that very quickly has a negative effect, both mentally and physically. If unrelieved, said the Daoists, this energy-overload brings on a variety of illnesses, ranging from headaches to hysteria, and also causes a great deal of the mental and physical violence that human beings inflict upon each other.

Contemporary scientific research has, in fact, corroborated these ancient Daoist beliefs to an impressive degree. There is growing evidence to indicate a direct relationship between violence and the frequency and quality of sexual activity among adults.

In societies where there are severe restraints on sexual behavior, extreme violence is commonplace. The tighter the sexual controls, the more violent the society tends to be.

Having discerned the relationship between sexual activity and health, this branch of Daoist philosophers began preaching that people should engage in sex two or three times a day when young and at least once a day from middle-age on.

More experience and observation led the Daoists to the obvious conclusion that older men function more effectively when their female partners are young, and that regular performance is further enhanced when there are a variety of partners as opposed to having the same one all the time.

In a burst of male generosity, it was also acknowledged by these Daoist wisemen that older women benefited from having young men as their sexual partners.

This particular school of Daoism experienced a significant increase in its popularity shortly after this new sexual philosophy was propounded, and soon spread to Japan. Given their traditional fertility rituals and overall appreciation of sex not only as a normal, natural function but also as an essential element in the scheme of life, the Japanese had no problem accepting this new import from China.

Of course, this new wrinkle in Daoism was not sanctioned for all Japanese. It was primarily the prerogative of those in power who, after all, were the ones with the time and means to enjoy such healthy measures.

Still, the concept spread far and wide and became woven into the fabric of Japanese culture. Along with Shintoism, it was to underpin the sexual mores of the ruling shoguns, provincial fief lords, and the large samurai warrior class during the long feudal period from A.D. 1192 to 1868.

CHAPTER 4

Happy Days of Hedonism

The sensuality of traditional Japanese culture culminated in the middle decades of the long Tokugawa Shogunate, (1603–1868) which is also known as the Edo period, after the great Edo Castle where the shogun lived and held court.

The more affluent men of this period had access to a variety and volume of sexual activity that has probably never been surpassed on a nationwide basis in any other country, before or since. (The shoguns themselves had huge harems.)

The Edo period also saw the rise of the geisha, the heyday of sanctioned red-light districts (the "floating worlds" of Japanese literature), hot baths featuring the sensual services of young women, and a vast national network of inns that also functioned as houses of assignation.

Perhaps the best-known of the institutionalized purveyors

of sensual pleasure were the geisha, who began as part entertainers, part prostitutes, and never escaped the reputation, whether deserved or not.

Within several decades after their first appearance and recognition as a specific class of entertainers, the geisha were organized. Girls recruited into the ranks, sometimes as young as nine or ten, were put through years of rigorous schooling in the art of entertaining men, including on-the-job training as dancers, singers, and players of the shamisen.

All geisha were sexually available to patrons in one way or another, but generally speaking, the higher class geisha did not work on a nightly or regular basis as prostitutes. They were expected to develop intimate relationships with favored patrons, however, and might have several in serial fashion. Less attractive geisha were often forced into semi-prostitution by their masters.

By the time Japan's last great shogunate was beginning to break up in the mid–1800s, the more beautiful and successful geisha were held in high esteem and were often taken as wives by successful men. Virtually all leading statesmen, politicians, and businessmen of this period had geisha mistresses, and this practice continued until World War II.

But it was the great red-light districts of the Edo period that set the tone for much of urban life in Japan from the late 1600s until the 1950s. Every town and city had one or more pleasure quarters. The most famous of all was Tokyo's *Yoshiwara*, which was known as the "Nightless City," and was the impetus and center for much of the cultural activity that flourished during this period.

This huge district, with its high walls, formidable gates,

and lantern-festooned streets, attracted sword-carrying samurai, merchants, priests in disguise, artists, writers, gamblers, sumo wrestlers, and others.

The *Yoshiwara* and the hundreds of other larger red-light districts had their own protocol and laws that were strictly enforced. A special language made up of a unique vocabulary and mode of expression developed within this "floating world."

There was a popular saying in Japan during this period that there could be no better fortune than to be a man and live in Edo.

Just as important and perhaps even more conspicuous in Japan's dedication to sexual release during the long, mostly peaceful Tokugawa Shogunate was the great chain of inns linking the country—inns that came about because of one of the most extraordinary political phenomena in the history of any nation.

When Iemitsu Tokugawa, grandson of Ieyasu Tokugawa, founder of the Tokugawa Shogunate, became shogun in the 1630s he established a political control system known as *Sankin Kotai* (Sahn-keen Koh-tie), under which some 250 of the nation's 270 fief lords, known as *daimyo* (die-m'yoh) or "Great Names," were required to build mansions in Edo, keep their families there at all times, and themselves spend every other year in the capital in attendance at the shogun's court.

This meant that every other year, each clan lord, along with a specifically prescribed retinue of samurai warriors, retainers, servants, and so forth, had to travel by foot from his domain to Edo, stopping each night along the way, and then return along the same route one year later. Those lords whose fiefs were in western Honshu and far-off Kyushu were therefore on the road for several weeks on each trip.

When the lord of the Maeda clan, the largest and richest of the fiefdoms, traveled to Edo his procession numbered approximately 10,000. One can imagine the sight and impact of this huge column of distinctly uniformed warriors and retainers as it passed through villages and towns along the way, stopping each night at a cluster of inns. (The Maeda lord maintained four mansions in Edo during the nearly 250 years this system remained in effect.)

As a result of this strictly enforced shogunate edict, the greatest network of traveler accommodations the world had ever seen sprang up almost overnight along the great walking roads that led to Edo from all over the country.

As the years of the Edo period rolled by, these huge "Processions of the Lords" were joined on Japan's roads by an increasing number of private and official travelers—messengers going to and from the shogun's castle and the Imperial Court in Kyoto as well as to the 270 clan headquarters, peddlers selling wares, merchants on business trips, gamblers, entertainers, ordinary people on religious pilgrimages, masterless samurai, and itinerant priests.

The larger of these roadside inns provided all the services male travelers normally expected—hot baths, food, bed, and female partners—there being no social or political sanctions against commercial sex. In fact, during this amazing period it was officially accepted as a matter of course that men away from home should not be deprived of regular sexual release.

Thus it came about that Japan, with its geisha, red-light districts, and extraordinary system of travelers' inns, came closer perhaps than any other country to providing sanctioned, institutionalized sexual outlets for a big percentage of its male population.

Of course, this was a system based absolutely on the chauvinistic attitude that men have sexual needs and women do not—or at least that the needs of women are not important enough to be given serious consideration.

Japanese men neatly sidestepped any moral dilemma by clearly distinguishing between ordinary women who did not engage in premarital or extramarital sex and those who did. Those who did were known as "public women."

This term generally applied to any woman who worked outside of her home, but particularly to those who worked in the entertainment, food, beverage, and accommodation industries, which eventually came to be known as the *mizu shobai* (mee-zoo show-bye) or the "water business."

About the only consolation Japanese women as a group might have had over the long centuries of their history is that some of them worked outside of their homes and were therefore eligible to exercise their sexuality—albeit not always when they wanted to or how they wanted to.

But the women of Japan were to have their day!

CHAPTER 5

Sampling Forbidden Fruit

When the first Westerners began arriving in Japan in the 16th century, they were immediately attracted to Japanese women. But most Japanese women regarded them as hairy barbarians and were afraid of them. The foreigners were, in fact, usually hairy and generally speaking had barbaric manners when compared to the strict, stylized etiquette of the Japanese.

Eventually, however, most of these men were able to take advantage of the Japanese customs regarding sexual behavior by consorting with recognized "public women." Interestingly, after Japanese women came to know the foreign visitors, and particularly after the foreign men learned that bathing regularly would not result in a lingering, painful death, intimate liaisons between foreign men and "non-public women," who could not resist the temptation, occasionally occurred.

The most interesting story of the reaction of Japanese women to foreign men during the early years of the Tokugawa Shogunate involved Dutch traders who were allowed to maintain an outpost on a tiny man-made island called *Deshima* (Day-she-mah) in Nagasaki Harbor after Japan closed its doors to the outside world in 1639.

The foreign traders were kept totally isolated on the islet except on very special occasions when they were escorted ashore by their samurai guards to pay their respects to the authorities and render gifts to officials.

Being humane if not kind, the Japanese authorities ordered that several Japanese prostitutes be rounded up every several days and escorted to the island for the Dutch to dally with.

At first, the girls selected for this duty had to be forcibly taken to the island, some of them bound to prevent them from escaping. They wanted nothing to do with those hairy barbarians who very closely resembled the terrible *tengu* (tane-guu) of Japanese legends.

The *tengu*, as every Japanese knew, were large, long-nosed, white-skinned, hairy wild men who lurked in the mountains and liked nothing better than to rape women and steal children. (I have always suspected that these legends were based on the possibility that long ago Western sailors had been ship-wrecked on the Japanese islands and survived for a while in the mountains.)

But within a remarkably short time, the prostitutes of Nagasaki completely reversed their attitude and behavior and began gambling for the opportunity to go to Deshima and do it with the Dutch. This system was continued for approximately 200 years. (Of course, both the traders and the girls were changed every few years.)

The fascination that foreign men had for Japanese women did not really become obvious until the 1860s when the Tokugawa Shogunate fell and foreign traders were allowed to take up residence in Yokohama, about twenty miles south of the shogunate capital of Edo (renamed Tokyo in 1871).

Just as the early Dutch traders had been kept isolated from the Japanese, the foreign community of Yokohama lived behind great walls that were constantly guarded by sword-carrying warriors.

Only a handful of Japanese had ever seen a Caucasian at this time, and people would line the street leading to the walled-off foreign community, hoping to catch a glimpse of one or more of them on the occasions when they were allowed to make short trips out of the compound. It was noted that most of these crowds were made up of women.

As time passed and the foreign community was allowed to mix socially with selected Japanese, a groupie phenomenon occurred. Some Japanese women were so fascinated by the foreign traders they began taking extraordinary measures and chances to spend time with them.

Comments made by some of the traders in correspondence of the time indicate that some women, especially the wives and daughters of higher officials, competed for the attentions of the more attractive foreign males to the point that a number of scandals occurred.

Apparently it was not only the exotic appearance and size of the foreign men that fascinated the Japanese women. The women were also attracted by the courtly, romantic behavior of the foreigners toward upperclass women—something they had never experienced or witnessed in their relations with Japanese men.

This phenomenon was, on a very small scale, just an inkling of what was to happen in Japan almost 100 years later.

CHAPTER 6

The Occupation Years
"West Mates East"

The United States Armed Forces, along with military contingents from World War II Allied Nations, ruled Japan from September 1945 until the spring of 1952. This action was known as "the Occupation of Japan," and was without a doubt the most remarkable military occupation of one country by another in the annals of history.

The first American Occupation troops arrived at Atsugi Air Base southwest of Tokyo on August 28, 1945, thirteen days after Japan's unconditional surrender.

After boarding trucks that they had brought along, the troops headed for Yokohama (where the man in charge of the Occupation, General Douglas MacArthur, was to set up temporary headquarters until preparations could be made for him in Tokyo). Shortly after leaving Atsugi, the convoy of

American troops was flagged down by a much smaller Japanese convoy carrying prostitutes whose services were immediately offered to the arriving American troops.

The Japanese instigators of the prostitute convoy believed that one of the first things the American troops would do in Japan would be to go on a rape rampage—something their own soldiers had done repeatedly in China, the Philippines, and elsewhere.

They wanted to protect their own women by taking the edge off of the lust-drive of the Americans. Of course, they had the right idea but both their timing and their approach was off, and much to their chagrin the American officers in charge of the arriving GIs not only turned them down they were rude about it.

Up to this point in Japan's history, the Japanese had lived in a Confucian-oriented society ruled over by a military dictatorship of one kind or another for nearly two thousand years. The people had obligations and duties but few rights. It was the law of the land that fathers ruled their families with absolute authority.

Virtually all marriages were arranged by parents or third parties, and romantic love was seen as an obstacle to the obligations of husbands and wives. Marriage was for the purpose of siring children and continuing the household; it was not an emotional affair.

Prior to the mid–1900s young unmarried Japanese men and women (with the very rare exceptions of those who had lived abroad and become Westernized), did not date in the Western sense.

Husbands and wives would visit family members together,

attend such public outings as cherry blossom viewings, and visit shrines or temples on special occasions, but as a rule they did not go out together—just the two of them—for social entertainment.

Married men who could afford to do so commonly kept mistresses, frequented houses of assignation—often with their wives' approval—and otherwise engaged in whatever extramarital activity took their fancy.

Young men who could afford to do so began visiting the red-light districts and/or assignation inns when they reached their late teens. For the most part, "non-public women" had no choice but to find other ways to sublimate their sex-energy buildup, or quietly suffer the consequences.

When the Occupation by foreign troops began, Japan's economy was shattered and the people, who had never known personal freedom before, were numb with shock and fright. They knew instinctively, from long historical experience, that the only way to survive a military defeat was to cooperate with the enemy, to adapt themselves to the new "winning lord;" to be passive and pleasing.

Fortunately for Japan, the "winning lord" was the United States—a country whose people had absolutely no affinity for war or the strict military occupation of an alien nation, especially one of which they knew virtually nothing, and whose people they could not communicate with or understand.

But what the Americans did have was a built-in compassion for people that surfaced almost immediately—an ability to quickly distinguish between the innocent civilian population of Japan and the arrogant military warlords who had started and pursued the war, and an inherent kindness that compelled them to begin immediately to treat the ordinary Japanese as victims who needed all the help they could get.

There was something else the newly arrived foreign troops in Japan had that was to influence the whole tenor and tone of the Occupation, and that was an immense reservoir of pent-up sexual energy—an aspect of the human condition that American society had traditionally ignored or down played as something that should not be recognized officially and preferably not even privately.

But away from home and in an alien society that was receptive to unbridled sexual activity, the bonds of American culture were easily slipped. As a result, an overwhelming majority of the Occupation forces were soon head-over-heels in an orgy of intercourse.

For perhaps as many as 70 percent of the young Americans it was their first experience with sex and they took to it with extraordinary alacrity.

Many factors beyond the sensual facet of Japanese culture contributed to this feast of ecstasy. The war had killed several million young Japanese men, leaving a significant imbalance between the sexes.

The war had also reduced most Japanese to living at a bare subsistence level, and the younger, more attractive women learned quickly that the foreign GIs, especially the always generous Americans, would shower them with food, clothing, money, and other amenities in exchange for sex and female companionship.

In no time, over two-thirds of all the male Occupationaires had full-time mistresses or were regular patrons at the newly enlivened red-light districts dotting the islands. The amount of money and goods pumped into the Japanese economy through this sexual link amounted to millions of dollars per month.

Hundreds of thousands of the women making up this link became serial mistresses, passed from one patron to the next as the GIs finished out their enlistments and were replaced by newly arrived troops.

The intelligence network of these women was incredible. They often knew well in advance—and often long before the Occupation personnel themselves knew—when individuals were going to be returned home or transferred to a new post in Japan.

On many occasions these young women would begin looking for new patrons weeks ahead. Sometimes the men who were leaving mistresses behind would help them find new patrons—often their own replacements. Some military personnel who had bought homes for their mistresses sold the homes to newly arrived replacements with the women willingly included in the deal.

Of course, a significant number of Occupationaires who took Japanese mistresses did not abandon them. They married them—often to the dismay of their families back home.

Partly as a result of the clamor caused by the growing number of GI-Japanese marriages, the military powers took considerable pains to discourage such unions. They made the process of applying for permission to marry Japanese women lengthy, tedious, and embarrassing.

While there was no morally valid reason for opposing some of these mixed marriages, there weré many that should not have taken place. In too many cases the individuals involved could not communicate with each other beyond an infantile and physical level. Often the GIs involved were poorly educated and of very low character.

In many cases the women were years older than their would-be spouses, had been working as prostitutes since their early teens, and were merely using the young, naive men to better themselves economically at the moment.

Oddly enough, a high percentage of the lower class men who married or applied for marriage to their Japanese girlfriends actually disliked the Japanese as a whole and had absolutely no affinity for the culture.

I had the extraordinary experience of being given the responsibility of interviewing military personnel assigned to one agency in Tokyo who applied to marry their Japanese girlfriends. My task was to discourage them; to talk them out of getting married.

I cannot remember how many servicemen I interviewed, but I do remember very clearly that I had no success whatsoever—not one. In one case, an extreme one in which the individual had been in Japan only three days when he put in for marriage, I succeeded in getting him transferred to Korea after he refused to even consider postponing his application.

The woman he wanted to marry was notorious. The only reason he gave, repeatedly, for wanting to marry her was that she was the best f... he'd ever had.

Stories about this mass meeting and mating of hundreds of thousands of American GIs and officers and Japanese women are endless. One of my own experiences that I will never forget: I stayed overnight at the home of a girlfriend one weekend (her mother liked me and approved).

The next morning, the 13-year-old sister of my girlfriend came into my bedroom and showed me an old "48 Position Sex Chart" that had been in the family for generations. She wanted me to point out my favorite positions. At that time, I thought I was pretty suave, but I blushed and stammered like I'd been caught behind the barn with my pants down.

One of the more imaginative Occupation escapades, pulled off by three corpsmen assigned to a Tokyo hospital, was the talk of the town for a while. They strung a curtain down the middle of their ambulance, hired two "working" girls to staff the "house on wheels," and drove around the city, soliciting business from foot-loose GIs.

Word was the experience was such a turn-on the enterprising trio built up a large number of repeat customers.

As usual where large concentrations of military personnel are concerned, the primary meeting points for liaisons with local women are bars that sprout in the vicinity. Japan was no exception.

There was one or more bar districts near every Occupation camp or post in the country. Each bar had a staff of girls as its main draw. Some bars had adjoining rooms for private use, but most of the trysting that resulted from the bar contacts took place in nearby inns or hotels.

Surprising to some, most Occupationaires did not patronize the many red-light districts throughout the country. The women working in these districts had had few if any foreign customers and generally spoke no English.

Most of the servicemen and civilian personnel assigned to Japan did not learn enough of the Japanese language to communicate on any level, and tended to frequent small places known as GI hang-outs, where the girls spoke some English.

Furthermore, having had little or no experience with red-light districts, Americans in particular did not feel comfortable in such large-scale institutionalized settings. Dealing with brothel madams, and knowing there were tough male "guards" lurking in the background, was pretty intimidating to the novice.

But above and beyond the lack of language ability and inexperience of the Occupationaires, most of the red-light districts (unless they were set up just for foreigners, such as one at Yokosuka Naval Base south of Tokyo), actively discouraged the GI trade.

Many of them totally barred foreign customers, including those who could speak Japanese, for the simple reason that they knew they would lose all of their Japanese trade if they allowed foreigners in—and they knew the foreigners would eventually disappear.

I recall visiting Gifu's famed "floating world" district in the summer of 1950. The buildings were all traditional inn-style, surrounded by garden landscaping complete with miniature rainbow bridges across flowing streams, huge stone pagoda-style lanterns, a forest of willow trees, and colorful paper lanterns strung on overhead lines.

The women, all dressed in bright kimono and wearing the polished *katsura* (kot-sue-rah) wigs, lined the curving walkways. It was a setting and a scene that had not changed for 200 or more years—and for those with an affinity for traditional Japanese culture, it was like a dream world. Despite being able to communicate fairly well, I and my friend were not admitted.

The Allied military occupation of Japan officially ended on April 28, 1952, but the American military presence there remained large and conspicuous for several additional years. The GI bars and assignation inns continued to flourish.

But by the summer of 1955, ten years after the end of the war, not only was the American presence shrinking at a visible pace, the Japanese were beginning to emerge from the background.

CHAPTER 7

The "Romance Gray" Phenomenon

As noted there was only limited courting and romance among the ordinary people of pre-World War II Japan—although it was common in feudal Japan at the courts of the emperor in Kyoto and the shogun in Edo (Tokyo).

One significant exception to the general rule of little or no courting among ordinary Japanese were romantic liaisons that developed between prostitutes and geisha and their special customers—liaisons that provided themes for many of Japan's famous literary works of that era as well as for more contemporary movies.

The reason such liaisons were more likely to involve "public" women is that generally speaking these were the only women with whom men could develop intimate relationships. Young unmarried men and non-public women spending time together, falling in love, and carrying on intimate relationships was contrary to the Japanese custom, and therefore rare. Those that did occur often ended in tragedy.

The political reforms imposed on Japan by the American-led Occupation Forces included freeing women from the tyranny of the Confucian family system and giving them the right to exercise more control over their own lives.

This, combined with the fact that the old male-dominated order in Japan had been totally discredited by the disastrous war and the fact that women were forced by necessity to play a key role in the recovery of Japan, laid the foundation for the rise in women's social, economic, and political status to levels previously not even imaginable.

It was the incredible influx of American culture into Japan, via the hundreds of thousands of Occupationaires, movies, magazines, and the sudden importance of the English language that was to provide both the impetus and the means for huge numbers of urban Japanese girls and women to take advantage of their new freedom, to break out of the steel cocoon they had been encased in for so many centuries.

Japan owes an immeasurable debt to the women who were teenagers in the 1940s, 50s, and 60s. It was they who led the changes that altered Japan from feudal monolith to the colorful menagerie it is today.

Not only did these young women begin wearing bright dresses, high heels, and make-up, they were the first sizable group to learn how to communicate in English and deal with foreigners. They were the first to resist the old arranged marriage system, to become hooked on American music, to begin changing Japan's eating habits, and to do so many other things that helped make Japan what it is today.

For an insular, proud, and often arrogant people like the Japanese to be utterly defeated in a war they started, and then to be occupied by an alien other-race enemy, had to have been one of the greatest cultural shocks any people could ever experience.

However, within the overall shock, the one facet that was perhaps the hardest for the older people to take—especially for the men to bear—was the daily and nightly sight of hundreds of thousands of Japanese women consorting openly and enthusiastically with foreign men. The fact that the foreign men were the former enemy made the taste even more bitter.

The emotional feelings this sight aroused were understandably intense, but amazingly, there was very little outward show of emotion by the majority of Japanese men and older women. Altercations between young Japanese men and foreign GIs, over women, were few and far between.

The public dating and displays of affection between the Occupationaires and their Japanese girlfriends were obviously irritating to an extraordinary degree, but the fact was the foreign men had not displaced Japanese men as partners for the Japanese women involved. They were doing things young Japanese men had never done in the first place.

And it was, perhaps, this cultural factor that kept the level of violent reaction very low. In fact, until well into the 1960s one of the first questions Japanese men typically asked newly arrived foreigners (sometimes before they had been in the country for a full day) was how they liked Japanese girls. One American movie star who was still in Tokyo's Haneda International Airport responded to this question by replying,

"I don't know. I haven't tried one yet!"

Even after Japanese men began picking up on the practice of dating "non-public" women in public, it was generally not the younger men as would normally be expected, but older married men—men who were in their 50s, 60s, and older.

The reason for this was very simple, very basic. Most young men, whether single or not, did not have the money to take women out to restaurants, theaters, resort inns, or other places where there was cost involved.

This phenomenon of young girls dating older men reached its peak in the mid–1950s, resulting in reams of newspaper and magazine hype and numerous movies with a "Romance Gray" theme, in reference to the fact that the men involved in these hundreds of thousands of liaisons were gray-haired. That was a golden time for older men with money in Japan!

And it was not only older Japanese men who created and took advantage of this sex-with-young women boom. Foreign men in fact were in the vanguard of the phenomenon. By this time (the mid–1950s) hostess cabarets, some of them on a huge scale, had appeared in Tokyo and other major cities throughout Japan. These cabarets were staffed by some of the most beautiful women in the country, and it was in these great cabarets that affluent foreign businessmen (who were flocking to Japan by the thousands to buy cheap goods) did most of their girl hunting.

Hundreds of these businessmen, some of whom came to Japan only twice a year, established mistresss relationships with girls they met at cabarets, and paid them thousands of dollars a year in living allowances and fees.

One hostess-mistress, who lived in the Yoyogi apartment

building where I lived, had two patrons, and used to regale us with stories about how she kept them apart when they both showed up in Tokyo at the same time. She said some of her friends had up to four out-of-country patrons.

Some of the foreign visitors ended up marrying their cabaret hostess-mistresses. Perhaps the most notable case of this was Sukarno, the president of Indonesia from 1945 to 1967. On an official visit to Tokyo he and his entourage put up at the Imperial Hotel. One of his aides was sent out to get some girls from a Ginza cabaret. Sukarno was so taken by the girl brought to him that he married her—setting a very high standard for other hostesses to follow.

The "Romance Gray" phenomenon was a news media and entertainment topic for nearly two years. The boom itself reached its peak in 1955/56 and then began petering out as the economy picked up speed and the incomes of both young men and non-public women continued to rise. The custom for older men to liaison with younger women, from both the entertainment trade and regular business, did not disappear, however.

In fact, as in other countries older men having sexual access to younger women was a well-established custom in Japan, going back to the beginning of its history. Upper class men had always been permitted to have concubines, who were invariably young. Affluent, powerful men also had mistresses, usually much younger than themselves. And it was almost always older, affluent men who were the chief clients of geisha and elite prostitutes.

This practice had just continued to evolve with the times. The "Romance Gray" boom was unique only in that the young women had a choice and *they* often took the initiative.

The other unique factor, of course, was that during this time there were large numbers of young, single Japanese men waiting on the sidelines, anxious to get onto the playing field for the first time in Japan's history.

CHAPTER 8

Love Hotels &
Massage Parlors

Soon after Japan regained its sovereignty in the spring of 1952 various women's groups began to lobby for the elimination of all legal and illegal red-light districts in the country.

A number of women who were elected to the Diet (also for the first time in Japan's modern history) were among the chief spokespeople for this campaign. One of their points was that Japan's image in the eyes of the civilized world was being damaged by the fact that prostitution was legal in the country, and that many women were more or less treated like slaves.

The topic quickly became a media event, and eventually the male members of the Diet acquiesced out of embarrassment. A law was passed banning the practice of organized prostitution. The law went into effect on April 1, 1956, with a one-year grace period for all the people in the prostitution business to get out of it.

There was very little immediate change but as the year wore on, more and more of the houses (which resembled small inns or hotels) converted to other businesses. Some of them temporarily became photo studios featuring nude models (this was common in the Shinjuku 2-chome district in west Tokyo); others became retail shops, real estate offices, and the like.

More than a dozen of the proprietors in Tokyo's great *Yoshiwara* district, in Asakusa, were eventually to opt for hot bath/massage parlors.

I and some friends went to both Shinjuku 2-chome and the *Yoshiwara* on the last legal night of the grace period. It brought back a lot of memories, but it was a sad sight. It was still cold. The streets were mostly empty. A great many of the doors were boarded shut and there were few lights. In some areas it was so quiet we could hear trash paper in the streets being rustled by the wind.

It was to be some years before these areas again became viable business districts, and during this transition period the ripple effect of the new law banning red-light districts, plus the rising standard of living and the entry of hundreds of thousands of Japanese men and women into the premarital and extramarital mating game, changed the whole picture of sex in Japan.

One of the first of the extraordinary changes that began sweeping Japan from about 1952 was the proliferation of hundreds of thousands of coffee shops—some little holes in the wall; others taking up several floors in large buildings. Every one of these new shops had some kind of decorative and/or entertainment theme that was foreign and exotic (at least to Japanese eyes).

Some coffee shops featured beautiful waitresses who rotated from station to station, like models on runways. Others featured jazz music; some aired chamber music. Some had closed-circuit telephones in every booth so male and female customers could meet "over the phone." The variety of coffee shops was almost endless.

This was before the appearance of modern high-rise office buildings with Western style meeting rooms and air-conditioning, so businessmen held their meetings in coffee shops—which were the first to introduce widespread air-conditioning in Japan.

In Tokyo and other large industrial cities, the average low- and middle-ranking executives in virtually every company spent from one to three hours every day in coffee shops. In the evenings, the coffee shops were jammed by young people, male and female, generally in groups separated by sex, but as the years passed, more and more by dating couples.

With their tiny homes, one-room apartments, and small jam-packed offices, the Japanese—except for wives with children and elderly people—spent a significant portion of their waking hours in coffee shops.

By 1955 a recognizable "coffee shop culture" had appeared and was masterfully chronicled for a magazine I edited by up-and-coming writer-author Donald Richie.

In later years, coffee shops offering private bedrooms to couples also appeared on the scene.

Along with this network of coffee shops, a type of "short-time" and over-night hotels, called "lov-tels" by the press (known today as "love hotels"), began appearing by the thousands. They materialized almost everywhere—in and near entertainment and restaurant districts, near major commuter railway terminals, even in the pocket residential areas that still existed in the central wards of major cities.

At first, the clientele of the ubiquitous love hotels were primarily love-starved businessmen using them as trysting places to consummate affairs with female office workers and cabaret hostesses.

Before long, newspapers began to report that businessmen were also taking ultra-liberated female college students to love hotels. Some of the female students were in "Romance Gray" relationships, while others were just seeking extra pocket money from generous older lovers.

Anyone out on the town after 11 p.m. during these years was used to seeing thousands of taxis and private chauffered-driven cars scurrying between cabarets and night clubs and the local love hotels.

As the whole social scene in Japan continued to metamorphose, young unmarried couples also began utilizing lov-tels, as did husbands and wives who had no privacy in homes or apartments shared with grandparents and children.

The number and popularity of love hotels continued to grow over the years, and today they remain a conspicuous and significant element of sex in Japan. The experienced observer can count upwards of a hundred love hotels alongside the freeway from Narita International Airport to downtown Tokyo.

Several of the best-known and most used love hotels in Tokyo are in the popular Akasaka and Roppongi entertainment-restaurant districts, where some of them often double as businessmen's hotels.

Another institution in Japan that had its roots in the ancient past, died down during the war years and then came back with a vengeance during Japan's economic recovery, was the combination hot bath/massage parlor. There are several hundreds of them in Tokyo alone.

The ancestors of the present-day parlors were shogunate era bathhouses that provided young women as attendants whose services for male bathers included various sexual ministrations.

The earliest postwar versions of these hot bath/massage parlors were still known as Turkish baths, but in the early 1980s the name of the parlors was officially changed from Turkish baths to "soaplands" because of complaints from members of the Turkish diplomatic corps stationed in Tokyo who did not appreciate the implications.

The only real difference in the present-day bath-and-massage parlors and those of yore is the architecture, decor, and prices. They come in various shapes and sizes, from inn-like structures to multi-storied Western buildings. They are set up more or less like hotels, with small private rooms that included a steam box, hot bath, massage bunk, and usually a dresser with mirror.

Each room is staffed by a female attendant (sometimes two) who steams, scrubs down, then massages the customer. The massage, often just perfunctory, generally leads to sexual services.

Although the AIDS scare of the mid–1980s put a dent in the soapland business for a while—many of them strictly banned foreign clientele, specifying in particular those with tattoos—it was soon business as usual and they seem to be holding their own. (The tattoo ban still exists in many places, however, including the new Edo-themed hot spring spa *Oedo Onsen Monogatari* (Oh-eh-doh Own-sen Moh-no-gah-tah-ree) on Odaiba, the man-made island in Tokyo Bay.)

While there are a few soaplands in Japan that are for women only, most of them are for men, and these are primarily men on the road—businessmen and other travelers who are in a city for just one, two, or a few nights, have no local connections, and no time or inclination to play the pick-up game in a bar or cabaret (which doesn't always work, and when it does, may be far more expensive than the soaplands).

In Tokyo and Osaka there are usually two or three soaplands that service foreign clientele exclusively or almost so. They have English-speaking attendants and often provide such amenities as copies of *Fortune* and the *Wall Street Journal* in their waiting rooms.

Unofficially, you can get soapland-type services in the privacy of your own room at some of the best-known hotels in Japan.

If I were to rate Japan's love facilities, all except a few of the more pretentious soaplands would come in on the bottom of the list. They do have their place, however. Besides being convenient they also feature one thing the Japanese have always associated with sex—a before and after hot bath.

The institution of the geisha still exists in Japan, and they are still patronized almost exclusively by leading politicians and businessmen (no one else can afford the cost). But their numbers have dwindled down to a few thousand. While there were dozens of famed geisha districts in Tokyo alone as recently as the 1960s, there are now just a few remaining.

CHAPTER 9

Porn for the Male Masses

In Japan's lexicon of love, pornography has traditionally played a significant role. But it has lost something in recent decades; something that can probably be traced to American style consumer-market influence.

Traditional Japanese pornography—graphic portrayals of sexual activity in all of its possible human ramifications—was generally stylized and artistic, drawn and painted with considerable skill. While the quality did not gainsay the subject matter, it did give some of the work a value of its own.

More importantly, however, given their sexual attitudes and customs, the Japanese did not look upon sexually explicit printed or carved materials as sinful or sleazy or dehumanizing or demeaning. They were generally not spread out on the tea table for visitors to admire (or be shocked at), but they too had their place.

In the case of the popular "sex position charts," they were often given to newly married couples on their wedding night. Notwithstanding the merriment and seeming embarrassment this invariably caused, the purpose was serious enough.

But the style, content, and purpose of Japan's postwar pornography is totally different from the traditional genre. It is first of all strictly commercial, with no redeeming social value that I can discern.

Japan's pornographers, just like Japanese producers in other product areas, have taken something someone else started and made it bigger and better (in a technical sense), by mass-producing it and developing a huge market where none existed before.

Most pornography in Japan today is produced in the form of black-and-white line drawings printed in comic magazine format, although there is also a substantial industry that produces photographic porn on high-gloss paper a la America's "sophisticated" men's magazines.

A key difference in porn in Japan and porn in the United States is that in Japan it is mass marketed to young boys as well as adult males and is absolutely everywhere. It can be bought in stores, shops, kiosks, and newsstands that are more common than hamburger shops, convenience markets, and drugstores in the United States

Perhaps the most interesting aspect of porn in Japan is that the people who buy it read it in public on buses, subways and trains, in coffee shops, snack bars, and elsewhere. Boys and men who read it in such public places make little or no effort to conceal it from the view of others.

Innumerable times I have been on crowded trains and subways next to someone reading fully illustrated comic-book porn that was equally visible to women young and old around them, obviously without feeling any sense of embarrassment or wrong-doing.

Surely the next most interesting facet of Japanese comic-book porn is that a great deal of it emphasizes the most extreme forms of sadism perpetrated on women. Scene after scene, page after page, story after story, depicts women being savagely assaulted and sexually violated.

There was, however, a softer, more romantic side to some of the porn that began to appear in the late 1980s. After millions of Japanese had traveled abroad to such places as Guam and Hawaii, a new kind of porn, aimed at young travelers, began to appear in a development that clearly revealed the commercial nature of the porn makers.

I first saw this new porn being read by a high school boy on a subway in Tokyo. The setting of the story was a yacht anchored off a tropical island. A group of boys and girls, who looked like they were in their mid-teens but were no doubt intended to portray high-teens, were on a scuba diving party.

The reason why the comic-book characters were made to look so young is that Japanese men are fascinated by girls with baby faces who look and act infantile, and use them in their sexual fantasies as well as their business advertising.

The story line was what one of the boys did to one of the girls while both were underwater. The compelling part, from my Western viewpoint, was the fact that the participants were made to look so young, and the excruciatingly funny expressions the artist drew on the face of the girl while she was being had and when she climaxed.

The thought that kept coming to my mind was that the comic would probably attract thousands more young boys and girls to go on scuba diving trips overseas.

Many Japanese publishers who are not mainline pornographers, and in fact are highly respected Establishment publishers, routinely add little porno featurettes to their magazines.

Since the Japanese do not react to pornography the way most Westerners do, the influence of this volume of mass-marketed pornography is probably different as well.

Looked at in the overall context of love and sex in Japan, the part that concerns me is the sadistic content of a great deal of it and what it might mean for Japanese women. At the same time, Japanese women themselves have not been overlooked as sexual consumers.

CHAPTER 10

Sex Lessons
for the Ladies

Japan has one of the most dynamic, diversified and daring publishing industries in the world. Most Japanese, and some non-Japanese as well, also regard it as the most advanced, not only economically but also in terms of concept, design, and marketing.

Magazine publishing is especially advanced, and not surprisingly includes the most aggressive publishers in the country.

A major reason for the extraordinary depth and diversity of publishing in Japan, particularly in areas that are culturally sensitive such as sex, is precisely because the Japanese have a different cultural background and therefore different values.

A society that condones the production and mass-marketing of sadistic pornography to its male youth is not likely to have any qualms about marketing explicit sexual materials to its young women, but with a difference, of course.

Since the male-oriented society of Japan has always distinguished between the sexes, with women treated as sex objects on the one hand and as the epitome of femininity and virginity on the other, male magazine publishers wanting to tap the rich female market simply adopted an educational approach.

By assuming the stance that Japanese women knew nothing about sex, and taking the high road that sex education was essential for them to become complete women, they justified a whole slew of magazines that both educate and titillate, to a degree that non-Japanese tend to regard as over-kill.

The Japanese attitude toward sexual matters can be both amusing and disappointing, especially where foreigners are concerned. I remember back in the early 1950s when the red-light districts were still flourishing and were a common topic of conversation. (I and virtually all other foreign men of my acquaintance were always being teased about going to the districts.)

When I brought the subject up, however, Japanese women would often deny that the sex centers existed. After a little pressure on my part to force them to admit the areas were really there, they would then insist that no Japanese men ever patronized the houses.

When I would point out that the districts had been in existence for decades to hundreds of years, long before the mass arrival of foreigners, they would then say that only gangsters went to the quarters.

This reaction was obviously an attempt to save face in the

front of foreigners, but it went beyond just that and was also part of the residue of the ancient myth, accepted by both men and women, that Japanese women are superior to other women and at the same time are so pure they know nothing of worldly things.

This attitude is often especially conspicuous where sex is concerned, when the contradiction between reality and myth is so direct, so overwhelming, it becomes ludicrous (to a Westerner). As when a young, sweet, charming girl will behave with absolutely angelic innocence, and then prove to be a master lover only moments later.

Of course, there is nothing dumb or devious about this attitude and behavior. It is one of the most potent sexual turn-ons known to man.

As for the sex magazines aimed at young unmarried women, the first ones began with a clinical approach (just as did America's women's magazines and television sex-talk shows), and then began to widen their scope as competition inevitably entered the picture. From then on, it was educate and titillate with no holds barred.

Some of the sexual advice being given to young Japanese girls today is enough to make your toes curl.

Just as in the comic-book porn produced for young Japanese men, Japan's sex-oriented women's magazines also illustrate their messages, primarily with line drawings, since these tend to make the illustrations impersonal and prevent any conflict with Japan's anti-pornography laws (which are primarily designed to keep foreign pornography out of Japan; not stem the home-grown industry).

By using line drawings, the sex magazine publishers can

make technical points about how to perform a wide variety of sexual activities, and get across other messages at the same time. Of course, this takes refined artistic skill, but the Japanese are world renowned for that kind of hands-on ability.

As mentioned earlier, the innocent cuteness that pervades so much of Japan's commercial advertising also appears in drawings of young people engaged in very sophisticated sex acts.

Again, this is a manifestation of Japan's traditional culture keeping up with the times, and cannot be compared with the gross character of some American and European porn magazines. No matter how "sinful" non-sadistic Japanese pornography may be in the eyes of Westerners, it is often done with a style and sense of humor that is, well, delightful.

What all of this printed sexual material means to love in Japan is obvious. It not only keeps people primed and ready and provides them with technical examples to experiment with and follow it also provides the philosophical and moral bed for lovers to lie in. That, it seems to me, is a worthwhile, even enviable, accomplishment.

CHAPTER 11

Titillation
On the Tube

Japanese acceptance of human sexuality from the beginning
of their history made it natural for them to treat television as
just another visual medium, essentially no different from the
stage or woodblock prints.

This meant that sexual subject matter and sexual scenes
were not automatically taboo. What happened, however,
is that Japan's television industry imposed some limits on
itself in deference to possible criticism from the international community. The same rationale that resulted in
banning legal prostitution also influenced TV programming
from the beginning.

This did not mean that TV programmers completely
eschewed the drawing power of sex. A society that celebrates
sexuality by joyously parading giant penis replicas through

the streets is not going to impose unrealistic restraints on a medium as marvelous as television.

One of Japan's most popular festivals depicts young men, with huge mock penises strapped to their groins, rushing into villages and attempting to have public intercourse with every young woman they can find.

The young women run about and try to hide behind their friends, but all the while squealing and laughing and enjoying the symbolic act as much or more than anyone else. This festival has often been shown on television.

Television comedy skits, starring well-known players, often feature on-screen "dry rapes" as part of the action, getting huge laughs from audiences. TV cameramen will often get down on the floor or follow young women upstairs, aiming their cameras under their dresses, in blatant examples of sex exploitation that draw no widespread rebukes, no mass protests by women's groups. It is treated as risque, but otherwise perfectly acceptable behavior that does no harm when beamed into millions of homes.

The Japanese do not regard nudity per se as either lewd or sexual. When the nudity is in a normal, natural setting, the nudity itself is perfectly normal and natural. It is normal for a person to be nude in a bedroom or bathroom, even when the bath is outside in public. Japanese television shows, particularly travel programs, will often show people, men and women, bathing together.

In fact, travel programs about hot spring spas where mixed bathing is the rule are among the most popular TV fare. In most of these, the host commentators are attractive young women who not only interview nude bathers, they strip (off camera) and join them, on camera.

Now this requires a degree of aplomb that probably few foreign television personalities have, and is something that they should view with envy. Certainly the ratings of some of them would improve if they did their thing in the buff.

Before anyone gets the idea that the Japanese are totally without modesty, it should be noted that both men and women bathers cover their genital areas with small hand towels when they are moving about outside of the water. Which means, of course, that viewers seldom see more than female breasts and lots of flesh. But just having a face cloth between you and millions of people still requires a substantial dash of panache.

For years late-night television in Japan featured programs that would have been classified as pornographic in the United States The films emphasized extraordinary violence, usually against women, and sexual activity that included just about everything except stark close-ups of penile penetration (the point that American television is rapidly approaching at the time of this writing).

Interestingly enough, however, Japan's producers of late-night TV fare, under increasing pressure from women's groups, drew back at this stage and reduced both the sadistic and sexual content of their programs.

They are now well behind American programs of the same genre, and this is one area where an American television will probably continue surging ahead of its Japanese counterparts.

While Japanese television was a key factor in shaping and sustaining attitudes toward sexual behavior among the generations born during the 1950s, 60s, and 70s, today it no longer has a major influence on changes taking place in male-female relations. It has been surpassed by the porn magazines and passed by real life.

Of course, TV continues to reflect Japan's underlying sexual mores and in doing so helps validate and perpetuate them. But given the psychology of the Japanese, their sex-rated television programs will probably follow the lead of American television.

As soon as we get to the point where we will tolerate prime-time hardcore TV pornography for the masses—not just for sex channel viewers—the Japanese will probably feel justified in doing the same thing.

This inevitable development got a big boost with the appearance of small hand-held devices in 2005 that made it possible for the public to download content anywhere anytime, as easy as accessing a cell phone call.

Naturally, pornographers were the first to take full advantage of this new technology.

CHAPTER 12

Musume
On the Make

For those who are not linguistically inclined *musume* (muu-sue-may) means "daughter." During the years that American military forces occupied Japan the word came to be used by Americans to mean "girl" or "girls" in a general sense. They, however, usually pronounced it "moose" and it sometimes had the same connotation as "piece."

The word that the Occupation troops should have used is *Ojo-san* (Oh-joe-sahn), which means something like "Honorable Young Lady," and is used in several ways—when asking someone if an offspring is female, when wanting to note that a particular female is unmarried, when addressing a young girl whose name you do not know—in which case it is like saying "Miss!"—and when wanting to distinguish between a "public" girl who works in the "water business" and an "upright" girl who may or may not live at home but is credited with being "a regular girl."

Given the difference in the old image of a "public" woman and an *Ojo-san* as perceived in the traditional sense, the designation of "Honorable Young Lady" is very important—although this difference has significantly diminished in Japan's more Americanized society.

Not surprisingly, as the reputation of "public women" has gone up the image of *Ojo-san* has gone down, becoming much less idealized and much more accurate, bringing them closer together.

As mentioned earlier, Japan's first significantly liberated women were those who chose to fraternize with foreign men soon after the Occupation of Japan began in 1945. These women were scorned and vilified by Establishment Japan as well as the majority of Japanese men.

To a considerable extent they became outcasts in their own society—much further out than the traditional "public women" who remained "Japanese" despite their low-class, working occupations.

Most of the women who became "traitors to Japan" by associating with foreigners suffered intensely from the usually subtle discrimination and ill-will that was directed toward them. But being set adrift by their own society forced them to become self-reliant and to take care of themselves. The more capable among them developed an independent spirit and personal capabilities that had previously been rare for Japanese women.

All during the 1950s and well into the 60s, the most beautiful, the most interesting, the sharpest and the most intelligent women in Japan were often in the "water business," selling their femininity, their wits, and their charm in a business that was cut-throat competitive.

Those who rose to the top ranks in the world of cabaret hostesses were remarkable women indeed, far more intelligent and capable than most of the businessmen who patronized them.

Fortunately, the traditional self-restraint of the Japanese limited the occasions when the "public women for foreigners" were subjected to verbal and physical abuse. Physical violence especially was rare and when it did occur it invariably involved men who were drunk or who were low-level hoods known as *chimpira* (cheem-pee-rah).

I remember strolling in the Dogen slope Shibuya section of Tokyo one evening with two foreign friends and the Japanese wife of one of them. As three *chimpira* coming down the slope drew closer to us, it became obvious to me that one of them was going to deliberately bump the Japanese lady in our party.

At the very last instant, the lady's husband, who was over six feet tall and weighed some 190 pounds, jabbed his right elbow forward, deflecting the *chimpira* away with a jolt that almost knocked him down. I was surprised at the incident, first that the *chimpira* would make a frontal attack on a woman under those circumstances, and second that the woman's husband had obviously also seen the attack coming and had countered it so effectively.

The equally surprised *chimpira*, shocked by the unexpected turn of events, bobbed his head in an automatic bow and said *"Domo,"* an apology, in a typically Japanese reaction.

Urban Japanese girls who were in their early teens in the 1950s were exposed to a great deal of the interplay between foreign men and older Japanese girls. They saw them together in theaters, on the streets, and on buses and trains. They also read lurid stories in weekly and monthly pulp magazines that milked the GI-Japanese girl angle for all the circulation they could get.

Young Japanese girls were also conditioned by American movies and other media to have a romantic image of foreign men. This was compounded by racial and cultural differences that made foreign men attractive and fascinating to them, as well as by the fact that during this early period, most foreign men in Japan, including even poor students, were relatively well off financially and liked to spend money on Japanese girls, a custom that had not yet developed among young Japanese men.

Generally speaking, however, it was not the poorer Japanese girls who were the most likely to succumb to the attractions of foreign men. It was the *Ojo-san* of the better-to-do families—girls who had enough discretionary money to dress better than most and to frequent places where they were the most likely to meet foreigners.

In Tokyo in particular there were a number of places that were noted for attracting Japanese girls on the prowl, including the Imperial Hotel and, during one period, the nearby Foreign Correspondents' Club. Like the group of women in the late 1800s who flocked to the foreign community in Yokohama and to foreign hangouts in those days, these young girls, like butterflies, flitted about, hoping that something exciting would happen to them.

For the most part, these young women were not overtly bold or aggressive and it was up to the foreign men who were present at the time to recognize the signs and respond to them.

This, of course, eliminated many of the men from the running. They simply didn't pick up on the cues or were not predatory enough to take advantage of the opportunities being presented to them.

During those years my circle of acquaintances and friends included some of the most sexually aggressive foreigners in Japan. The behavior of some of them was outrageous, but few of them did anything to anyone who did not knowingly put themselves in an intimate situation where the result was a foregone conclusion.

Probably the most outrageous—and successful—Lothario of all was a man who conducted most of his trysts in his car, in mid-day, while parked in front of the National Diet Building and other notable locations in central Tokyo while on his lunch break.

As the years passed and the Japanese became richer and more confident, the number of *Ojo-san* attracted to foreign men grew in proportion, as did the number of places where liaisons were initiated. This growing group of young Japanese women widened to include students, artists, music buffs, and others in general.

Meeting places expanded from hotel coffee shops and lobbies to "conversation" bars and coffee shops, and finally to discos.

Another phenomenon that began in the 1960s and has picked up momentum ever since is liaisons and marriages between foreign women and Japanese men—something that was previously rare. In fact, by the end of the 1960s the number of Japanese men marrying foreign women exceeded the number of foreign men marrying Japanese women, and it has continued to do so ever since.

The reasons for this phenomenon are diverse. Japanese men have never had the reputation of making "good" husbands in the Western sense. Neither have Japanese men been noted for being handsome by foreign standards.

Furthermore, while foreign men who marry Japanese women are not automatically expected to "become" Japanese to any degree at all, foreign women taking Japanese husbands invariably have to adapt themselves to some extent, especially if they live in Japan.

Economics surely plays some role in Caucasian women-Japanese men marriages, but certainly not in all of them. It seems to me that the basic answer lies in the personal experiences and psychology of the individual women concerned, particularly in their attitude toward Japan and Japanese culture, their affinity for the language and so on.

I have known dozens of such couples. Some of the foreign women concerned were my university classmates and co-workers in Tokyo in the 1950s and I count them as good friends. But I am not qualified to go beyond some very general statements.

In any event, the world of foreign women married to Japanese men is different enough that they have formed support groups.

Foreign women wanting to marry Japanese men will surely have more and more opportunities to do so as more Japanese men travel and live abroad and become more international in their outlook.

A major factor in this phenomenon has been the growing degree of self-confidence in Japanese men. In early periods the average Japanese male felt intimidated by foreign women, and professed to hold them in very low regard. Besides being physically big, the stereotype was that foreign women were loud-mouthed, lazy, unskilled in any of the finer arts, immoral, and looked down on all Asian men.

At the same time, a great many Japanese men traveling abroad had one very special goal: to sample a foreign woman. "Sex tours" for Japanese men have been big business since the early 1960s. In this case, the inferiority complex that usually limited the development of intimate relations with foreign women generally did not apply.

Japanese men were old hands at dealing with any woman, regardless of size, shape, color or character, as long as they were buying her sexual services and were in a dominant position.

Getting outside of the shell of Japan and learning that foreign women are women first and foreign second, a growing number of Japanese men are learning that the old image of foreign women is often wrong, and that they can develop close, satisfying relationships with them.

This is giving more and more of them the opportunity to be as courageous and as "non-Japanese" as Japanese women often are, and to express their membership in the "human race" as opposed to the ancient, narrow image of themselves as either not good enough to marry outside of the Japanese race or too good to marry out of it, depending on which of their complexes is in play.

The feeling of uniqueness that has been characteristic of both Japanese men and women since ancient times is still very strong. At the same time, there is a growing desire to be less Japanese in the narrow, negative sense—to prove to themselves and others that they are the equal of and acceptable to people outside of Japan. The strongest way these feelings can be expressed is often sexual.

This suggests that the number of *Ojo-san* on the make for that ultimate foreign experience will continue to grow, and that young Japanese men who want to add their bit to international relations by taking foreign wives will also expand.

CHAPTER 13

When Hubby is Away, Wives Will . . .

There is one other important area of sex in Japan that I have not touched upon at all. Namely, the hundreds of thousands of Japanese wives, particularly those in their 30s and 40s, whose husbands are stationed away from home by their companies or who follow the traditional custom of leaving their wives pretty much alone and having most of their sexual recreation outside the home.

In the old days, the wives of common men generally accepted this kind of situation as a woman's unhappy lot in life. They were left to smolder, and when they became mothers-in-law, to take their frustrations out on their daughters-in-law.

Upperclass women of the ruling elite, including the numerous ladies-in-waiting at the courts of the emperor and shogun, often exercised their advantage of freedom from daily labor and other obligations to make and consummate love relationships with the husbands of their own class as well as raunchy priests and bachelors who had access to their circle.

Such liaisons are voluminously recorded in diaries written during Japan's long feudal period when the country was divided into some 270 fiefs ruled over by lords, who, like the shogun and emperor, had their own courts on a smaller scale.

One obvious reason for the volume of these affairs was, of course, that virtually all marriages, especially among the upper classes, were arranged and there were no emotional bonds between husbands and wives. Other obvious reasons were the corollary customs of concubines, mistresses, red-light districts, and unbridled hanky-panky offered to travelers on the road.

Given these traditions, which were legally as well as socially sanctioned until the middle of the 20th century, the propensity for a significant percentage of Japan's lonely wives to try to add a little love to their lives is readily understandable.

In the 1970s this situation saw the appearance of male-host bars and clubs that catered to married women of all ages. Many of the matron patrons of these places were well-to-do, and showered their host paramours with money, expensive clothing and trips abroad.

Still today, rumor has it that wives trysting with lovers are so common one can hardly shake a love hotel or hot spring resort inn without dozens of them tumbling out of bed. It is hard to make any kind of precise measurement of numbers, but there is no doubt that the figures are impressive.

A new factor in this aspect of male-female relations in Japan is that middle-aged married women now have the freedom, the opportunity, and the money to indulge themselves in all kinds of luxuries and special services, including those of the most intimate nature, if they are so inclined.

Most Japanese wives who are butterflying obviously do so with Japanese partners, but there are some with ties to the foreign community who have foreign lovers. Among these women are some who had their first foreign fling when they were young, before marriage. Some of them are wealthy jet-setters, well-known in Tokyo's business and diplomatic circles.

Fortunately or unfortunately, whichever the case may be, not many foreign men in Japan have the skills, means, or will to carry off affairs on this level, so this playing field does not represent a significant opportunity for foreign men seeking to broaden their experience in Japan.

No need for concern, however, as there are plenty of other opportunities.

CHAPTER 14

The Charms
Of Japanese Women

It is well established that foreign men find young Japanese women sexually attractive. It goes without saying that this attraction is physical and cultural, with both factors playing a very important role.

Although Japanese girls start out with the advantage of having a well-known reputation for making good wives and knowing how to please men, the obvious first stage in their appeal to foreign men is physical. A significant part of this physical appeal of Japanese girls is that they are small in stature, usually slender in build, and feminine in overall appearance.

Generally speaking, men are attracted to women who are smaller and weaker than they are. This means the women represent no physical threat, and reassures the man that if need be he can physically overpower the woman in order to have his sexual way with her. Small women make men fell bigger and stronger and more macho.

In watching foreign men interact with Japanese girls on hundreds of occasions, one of the most common things I've observed is for the men to put their hands up against those of the girls, and glory in the difference in their respective sizes.

The oohs and aahs of the girls really turn men on. In some raunchier situations (such as in cabarets) the girls will come right out and say with enthusiastic delight that the man's *musuko* (muu-sue-koe) or "son"—a common euphemism for the male organ—must be equally huge. . . which, of course, was the indirect intent of the comparison in the first place.

Men no doubt have other subconscious motives for reacting positively and sexually to smaller women. Of course, there is the very powerful motivation that smaller women "should" have smaller vaginas, reducing the possibility that the men will feel inadequate and shamed. Altogether, the petite stature of Japanese girls gives them a leg up on many of their foreign counterparts.

Another physical factor that plays a smaller but still interesting role in the attraction of Japanese girls is that when young they frequently have baby faces and look younger (to Western eyes) than their true age. This is another turn-on, and doesn't need any explanation.

The traditional almond-shaped eyes of Japanese (and other Oriental) girls is also a definite plus. Physiognomists tell us that curved eyes are, first of all, more beautiful than round eyes, that they are more sensual than round eyes, and that they impart a strong aura of mystery and seductiveness that raises male cockles.

There are, of course, extraordinarily beautiful Japanese women but they are in fact not common. Young Japanese women who are attractive would more often be properly described as cute rather than as beautiful.

The Japanese, like Americans, appear to have been mongrelized from a variety of races and to have produced a very high percentage of people who simply are not attractive. Fortunately for both, however, ugly parents do sometimes have beautiful children (it seems that nature favors the beautiful and strives to achieve it no matter what the obstacles). But the point here is that it is not the beauty of Japanese girls that attracts foreign males.

No doubt just as important as the petite figures of Japanese girls is their attitude and behavior. Their normal behavior, despite recent changes, is "feminine." This includes the way they move and talk, the way they dress, their general deportment. In social situations, and again despite a strong Western influence, Japanese girls generally conduct themselves according to traditional rules of etiquette that are very refined and very feminine when compared to typical Western behavior.

Where men and sex are concerned, Japanese girls have absorbed by osmosis a specific type of cultural behavior that pleases men. And not by coincidence or accident, of course.

A major part of the world of Japanese women has traditionally been concerned with how to please men. Included in this list of traditional cultural attributes are a number of things that many foreign women are likely to reject out-of-hand—behaving in a passive, subservient manner, catering to men, and so on.

Even when only a touch of traditional Japanese etiquette remains, it is still enough to set young Japanese women apart and make them appear especially seductive to foreign men (whose imagination also no doubt magnifies their attraction).

As we have already learned, Japanese girls do not have religious guilt hangups about sex. This makes them a lot more spontaneous and natural in their reaction to sexual situations. This is not to say that all Japanese girls are sexually promiscuous. Far from it. There are some, of course, who are as loose as they come, but the typical girl has very romantic notions and high standards, and must be romanced.

This romancing takes time and money and some skill, but once that is settled, sex comes naturally. And in this department, Japanese girls have some two thousand years of accumulated knowledge and a lot of contemporary advice on the variety of things two people can do and how to do them.

Other facets of love in Japan include the extraordinary support facilities in the form of the plentiful love hotels, the thousands of hot spring spa inns—mostly located in incredibly beautiful places along the seashores and in the mountains—that add a special touch to romantic assignations, and the equally extraordinary variety and number of restaurants and coffee shops that are designed to be romantic places where couples may meet and court.

In other words, Japan has commercialized, to a greater extent than any other country it seems to me, the sexual aspects of male-female relations, turning them into one of the largest and most profitable segments of their national economy.

Foreigners wanting to sample the Japanese love course should, however, keep in mind that there are some hazards that go with the game.

CHAPTER 15

The Wiles
Of Japanese Women

The same traditions that help make Japanese women good lovers also provides them with a great deal of power over men, if they choose to use it. Interestingly enough, it is usually only lovers and mistresses who routinely use this power. Once a girl becomes a wife, she tends to adopt another mode and base the relationship with her husband on other things.

Japanese women know from long experience that men lose some of their capacity to think rationally when they are sexually aroused (from whence my saying "hard on the bottom, soft on top" comes). When they want something from a lover, they will often use this knowledge, getting a man up and then not bringing him down until they get what they want.

Japanese women also know that one of the easiest ways to keep a man on a leash is to keep him drained of sexual energy.

He is not only much less likely to stray, he is less likely to even think about it. They use this knowledge to help them keep lovers and patrons in agreeable, docile moods.

Of course, some of the incentive for this is that they are very much aware that in Japan men have other choices.

Knowing how to exhibit sensuality and be seductive is another of the cultural skills of most Japanese women, and one they regularly use to attract and hold men. This does not require the exposure of a lot of flesh. In fact, truly wise women almost never expose themselves because mystery is far more tantalizing than open display.

The kimono and *yukata* (yuu-kah-tah) have traditionally been one of the prime weapons used by women to seduce male prey. They cover the wearer from neck to ankle, and yet attract men like flowers do bees.

Un-Westernized Japanese women also have the ability to exude a kind of innocent yet sensual vulnerability that affects some foreign men like a magic potion.

Like the legendary women who cry tears that turn men into obedient slaves, Japanese girls often resort to this weapon when things are not going their way.

One universal technique single Japanese girls use to get and keep men is to become intimate with them and then let friends and relatives know about the relationship.

This is especially effective where young foreign men are concerned, especially American men, because they are usually not sophisticated or experienced enough to deal with this kind of situation.

More than one young foreign man who has shacked up with a Japanese girl without any serious intentions has ended up marrying her after she invited her mother and later other members of her family to their love den, in effect putting the official seal on the relationship.

If the girl's mother actually ends up spending the night with her daughter and "practicing son-in-law" the young man might as well hang up his jockstrap. The final nail is often when the old man himself, the girl's father, is brought into the circle.

Of course, a growing number of young women in Japan have become Westernized to the extent that they no longer behave in the traditional Japanese fashion. Where contact and intercourse with foreigners are concerned, they are much more direct and open, and do such foreign-like things as curse, shout, and throw things.

Foreign men who get involved with this growing category of Japanese women should keep in mind that any violent behavior that might result will not necessarily take a form they are familiar with.

The most shocking case that came to my attention involved a man who arrived in Japan by himself, told a girl he was single and began living with her. A few months later he sprung the news that his wife and children were arriving and the girl would have to get out.

That night the girl encouraged the man to drink. After he went to sleep she got a butcher knife from the kitchen and chopped his penis off. Justice in the biblical sense, you might say.

CHAPTER 16

Look
Before You Leap

Stereotypes and prejudices die hard. Japanese men still believe that Japanese women make the world's best wives, that they are the hardest working, the best with children, the kindest, the most generous, and the most tolerant of their husbands, including any outside sexual adventures the husbands may have.

Of course, this is not true now and has never been true in a general sense. Most Japanese men simply do not know any better, and the claim merely shows their ignorance of the world at large.

There are many societies where the women as a rule are kind, generous, hardworking, and tolerant of husbands who are often lazy louts; some of them even accepting polygamous behavior by their men.

It is no doubt true that during Japan's long feudal age, most Japanese women were virtual saints, sacrificing their lives in a society made to serve male ambitions and idiocies, very much as women did in other parts of the world.

But young Japanese women today, particularly those in the major cities, are so different from past generations they (and young men) are often referred to as "new human beings," which, for the most part, means they are not "Japanese" in the traditional sense.

Still there is a quality about the typical young Japanese woman that, even today, sets her apart and makes her attractive both as a lover and as a wife. This quality includes a clear perception of herself as a woman who has her own place in the world and does not have to compete directly with men; along with a heightened sense of femininity and sensuality.

Among the things foreign men should keep in mind when contemplating the attractions of young Japanese women is that: (1) they tend to change more than American or European women do after they get married; (2) that if they are removed from the Japanese environment they tend to very rapidly lose some or all of the "Japanese" qualities that made them different in the first place; and (3) that long exposure to foreigners even in Japan has the same effect on a reduced scale.

Of course, these changes are not necessarily bad or undesirable. The more "Japanese" a girl is the more she *must* change if she is going to keep company with a foreign man, anywhere. The foreigner is not going to start acting Japanese, and a significant proportion of typical Japanese behavior by a girl friend or a wife is not compatible with foreign behavior, so as mentioned earlier, it is the woman who changes.

The obvious ideal situation for many foreign men in Japan, and one that is still common, is for them to enjoy the special attractions and talents of Japanese girls in their own natural habitat without forming the close, long-term relationships that result in them being foreignized.

Foreign women wanting to develop personal relationships with Japanese men are likely to take the opposite approach— that is, look for men who have already become less "Japanese" and who, in turn, are looking for what to them is the quintessential foreign experience—a sexual relationship with a non-Japanese, preferably Caucasian, woman.

The presumption here, of course, is that Japanese men without foreign experience or foreign language ability are not likely to aggressively pursue or be caught by foreign women—unless the women have become Japanized and would fit into the world of the "pure" Japanese male.

The main thing to keep in mind is that as exciting and satisfying as foreign-Japanese love affairs may be, they can also be more complicated and require extraordinary compensations and even sacrifices by one or both of the parties concerned if they "get serious."

Beyond this, about the only guidelines that I can suggest are: be honest and candid about your intentions; be considerate and discreet in your behavior; be firm and consistent in maintaining the relationship on the level intended; give advance notice, in a casual, controlled manner, when you decide to leave or go on to other affairs.

While it may strike some as being cynical and selfish, the most successful lovers I have known were those who always made sure they had an absolute minimum of two affairs going simultaneously and that their respective paramours knew about the other affair.

CHAPTER 17

Happy
Hunting Grounds

The "hunting grounds" for single men and women in Japan today—as well as for those who are married and still on the make—are not that different from those in the United States and other Western countries.

They include the usual places where males meet females—in school, at work, at outings of various kinds especially when groups are involved, through introductions from friends, at night clubs and other entertainment facilities, at cafes, and so on.

And just as in other countries, and over and above introductions, most relationships begin with males taking the initiative in meeting women whom they find attractive and going through the usual steps in establishing a relationship with those who are receptive.

Japanese women, like most women everywhere, are naturally skilled in letting men know they are interested and approachable. When Japanese women are not interested in particular men, they are equally skilled at ignoring them.

What makes the male-female game in Japan especially interesting and exciting for foreign males is not only the already mentioned exotic and seductive elements that are involved in the appearance and behavior of young Japanese women.

There is also the sensual wearing apparel favored by girls and young women, the fact that typical young girls and women are always well-groomed when they are out in public, and finally because there are so many of them in a very limited space.

Standing in one spot in one of Japan's thousands of entertainment and shopping districts, or in front of one of the dozens of thousands of busy commuter train stations, the stream of attractive young women going by is virtually endless.

There are, however, particular places in Tokyo and other Japanese cities where girl-watching is unsurpassed. The foreign male is not likely to meet any of these passing girls unless he is especially aggressive, but it will certainly whet his appetite.

Here are just a few of the more popular places in Tokyo where single girls and young women flock in large numbers:

1) The Ginza. This famous shopping, dining and entertainment district in downtown Tokyo attracts as many as a million people during the course of a single day and evening. Its boutiques and restaurants are a mecca for large numbers of the most stylishly dressed and attractive women in the city. The combined shopping/entertainment district boasts one of the largest collections of high-class bars, cabarets, and restaurants in all of Japan and is priced accordingly. This is one of the places that upper-echelon businessmen and politicians on expense accounts go to power drink and look for playmates.

2) Hibiya/Yurakucho (He-be-yah/Yuu-rah-kuu-choh). The attractions in these two small areas, which adjoin the Ginza on the west side, include an amazing selection of shops, restaurants, karaoke lounges, ballroom dance halls, pubs, cinemas, and the famous Takarazuka Theater which features all-girl revues that attract long lines of young girls waiting to get into the theater or to get the autographs of their favorite female performers.

3) Roppongi (Rope-pong-ghee). This is the favorite night-time hangout of single men and women who are into the bar, cabaret and night club scene, including foreign and Japanese movie and television stars, fashion models, rich playboys and young women who are attracted to all of the above.

Roppongi Intersection is the International Times Square of Tokyo. Japanese and foreigners alike begin massing here in the evening. By 8 p.m. the entire two-by-twelve block area resembles Ground Zero of a citywide party. Its hundreds of restaurants, bars, and discos are packed long after Tokyo's other entertainment districts have rolled up the sidewalks and turned out the lights. When young Japanese women want to meet "tall, sophisticated foreigners," whether just to live dangerously or to actually have a foreign romance, they go to Roppongi.

4) Shibuya (She-buu-ya). This famous dining and shopping center is especially popular with the young, and is noted for its boutiques that cater to teenage girls and women in their twenties. The statue of a dog (named Hachiko) in the plaza of Shibuya Station is one of the favorite rendezvous spots in the city.

In the evenings and on holidays and weekends, swarms of students and young people descend upon Shibuya like the great passenger pigeon flocks that used to cover several square miles in middle America. The attractions and prices in Shibuya's entertainment sections are geared toward the young and the young-at-heart.

5) **Aoyama-Harajuku** (Ah-oh-yah-mah/Hah-rah-juu-kuu). These two adjoining areas began as fashion centers and quickly developed into meccas for the young and trendy. The main thoroughfares are lined with boutiques, restaurants, cafes, and food stalls that give them a high-toned boardwalk atmosphere. On evenings and weekends Harajuku especially is jammed with people, including foreigners, absorbing the ambiance and looking for a good time.

6) Nishi-Azabu (Nee-she Ah-zah-buu). This relatively new entertainment area, just off the main thoroughfare that goes from Kasumicho to Hiroo, is made up of bars and restaurants strung out along what some people call "French Restaurant Row." The smallish, intimate French-styled restaurants attract a regular clientele of well-to-do, sophisticated women in their late 20s and 30s who respond to the international, romantic mood.

7) **Shinjuku** (Sheen-juu-kuu). The Kabuki-cho area of Shinjuku is either the armpit of Tokyo or the hottest entertainment district in town, depending on how you look at it. Bars, cabarets, clubs, love hotels, massage parlors, restaurants, strip shows, live porno acts...you name it and Shinjuku has it. Kabuki-cho, a few blocks north of Shinjuku Station, is often described as the sleaze capital of the city.

Despite the fact that most of the night-life businesses in Kabuki-cho are owned and operated by Japan's *yakuza* (yah-kuu-zah) gangster elements and foreign gangs that have entrenched themselves, the place is as safe as Sunday school as long as you stay out of the more obvious dives. The street drug-sellers and hoods who thronged the area in earlier decades have long since been eradicated.

Although its facade is now tame, step behind any of a thousand doors in Kabuki-cho and you are in the underworld of Tokyo's night life.

There is a large concentration of gay and transvestite bars in the 2-chome area of Shinjuku. The so-called *Golden Gai* is a collection of tiny *nomiya* (no-me yah), or drinking places, where you often need an introduction to get in. The list goes on.

More about Love Hotels
Most love hotels are immediately recognizable either because of their location in or near entertainment districts or in other areas where no regular hotel should be—or because of their conspicuous design.

For some reason love hotel operators like the castle or fortress look, and many opt for this style. Others are futuristic.

Regardless of their exteriors, the more pretentious lov-tels offer a variety of bedroom designs and furnishings. These range from ordinary undulating beds to beds made to resemble boats and cars, and such theme settings as Arabic harems to jungle hideaways. Many rooms also feature a variety of electronic gadgets and conveniences.

Rooms in lov-tels are rented by the hour, with a two-hour minimum until 10 p.m. After that the all-night charge applies even when you want the room only for a short time. Rates vary from YMCA to first-class hotel levels.

Lov-tels are the soul of discretion. There is usually no lobby; just a small curtained window where you pay in advance. Types of rooms are described in brochures available at the check-in windows and other distribution points, and on signs posted near the windows.

Most of Japan's large number of so-called businessmen's hotels also function as all-night lov-tels but without any special designs or gadgets. These may be best-suited for the foreign visitor or resident since no special knowledge is required, the clerks invariably speak enough English to get the job done, and their rates are reasonable.

Businessmen's hotels are listed in the local Yellow Pages and advertise in the English language media.

CHAPTER 18

Lover's Language

A

Abortion—*Orosu* (Oh-roe-sue).
Abortions are illegal in Japan, but are quite common because they are allowed if the pregnant girl or woman signs a statement saying that having a child would be detrimental to her physical or mental health, or would cause her financial difficulties.

She has had two abortions.
Kanojo wa aka-chan wo nido oroshimashita
(Kah-no-joe wah ah-kah-chahn oh nee-doe oh-roe-she-
mahsh-tah)

AC-DC, bisexual—*Nito-Ryu* (Nee-toe-R'yuu).
The *nito-ryu* was originally started by the famous swordsman Miyamoto Musashi, who used two swords, one in each hand, when fighting.

He is bisexual.
Kare wa nito-ryu desu
(Kah-ray wah nee-toe-r'yuu dess).

Acquainted—*Shiriau* (She-ree-ow).

I would like to get acquainted with that girl.
Boku wa ano onnanoko to shiri-aitai desu
(Boe-kuu wah ah-no own-nah-no-koe toe
she-ree-aye-tie dess).

Adult movies—*Poruno eiga* (Poe-rue-no a-ee-gah).
From the English word "pornography." Also *iro eiga* (ee-roe a-ee-gah) and *pinku fuirumu* (peen-kuu fu-ee-ruu-muu), "color" movies and "pink" movies respectively, both of which are used in reference to sex films.

Affair—*Yoromeku* (Yoe-roe-may-kuu).

She is having an affair with a young man.
Kanojo wa wakai otoko ni yoromeite iru
(Kah-no-joe wah wah-kie oh-toe-koe nee yoe-roe-may-e-
tay ee-rue).

Affected—*Kizappoi* (Kee-zah-poi).

He acts too affected.
Kare wa kizappoi desu
(Kah-ray wah kee-zah-poi dess).

Alimony—*Tegirekin* (Tay-ghee-ray-keen).
This literally means "hand-cutting money," which is pretty expressive, and refers to money paid in a lump sum in the form of a "buy-out." This kind of payment can be quite large, amounting to millions of yen in the case of a well-to-do man divorcing a wife. Monthly alimony is *fujoryo* (fuu-joe-rio). If a man has a child by a mistress he may be required to pay *yoiku hi* (yoe-ee-kuu hee) or "educational expenses" to the child's mother.

Amorous—*Iroppoi* (E-rope-poi).

He is a very amorous man.
Kare wa taihen iroppoi otoko desu.
(Kah-ray wah tie-hane e-rope-poi oh-toe-koe dess).

Amorous glance—*Netsuppoi metsuki* (Nate-sue-poi mates-kee).

That girl just gave me a sexy (amorous) look.
Ano onna-no-ko wa boku ni iroppoi metsuki wo shimashita
(Ah-no own-nah-no-koe wah boe-kuu nee e-rope-poi mates-kee oh she-mahsh-tah).

Also, *iroppoi metsuki* (e-rope-poi mates-kee), sexy look.

Arranged marriage—*Miai kekkon* (Me-aye keck-kone).
In pre-World War II Japan, most marriages were arranged by the parents or third parties, including professional marriage agents called *nakodo* (nah-koe-doe) or "go-betweens." The would-be bride and groom would see each other only once, twice, or maybe three times for brief chaperoned periods prior to the wedding. Young people in Japan today have a choice, and most marriages are *renai kekkon* (ren-aye keck-kone) or "love marriages."

Artificial virgin—*Jinko shojo* (Jeen-koe show-joe).
With the growth of plastic surgery in Japan in the early 1960s, one enterprising doctor came up with the idea of "restoring" the "virginity" of women who wanted to get out of the sex-for-sale business and get married. The new made-in-Japan maidenheads were an instant success, and dozens of other doctors began offering the same service. The technique involves reconstructing the maidenhead from remnants or from light plastic, which is sewn into place. Such new virgins were also called *shojo maku saisei* (show-joe mah-kuu sie-say), which literally means "virgin layer remade."

Attractive—*Miryoku-teki* (Mee-rio-kuu tay-kee).

You are a very attractive woman.
Anata wa taihen miryokuteki na onna desu.
(Ah-nah-tah wah tie-hane mee-rio-kuu tay-kee nah own-nah dess).

Slang terms used to express the same idea: *iitama* (ee-tah-mah), and *iisuke* (ee-sue-kay)

Attractive man—*Bidanshi* (Bee-dahn-she).

In Japan attractive men have many chances to philander.
Nihon de bidanshi wa uwaki no chansu ga takusan arimasu
(Nee-hoan day bee-dahn-she wah uu-wah-kee no chahn-sue
gab tock-sahn ah-ree-mahss).

Atami—*Atami* (Ah-tah-me).
This is a famous seaside hot spring spa about one hour south
of Tokyo, popular as a honeymoon and trysting place.

Let's go to *Atami*!
Atami ni ikimasho!
(Ah-tah-me nee ee-kee-mah-show!).

It is also a popular destination for year-end company parties,
especially because of its large number of "instant geisha" with
whom "one-night love" can be easily arranged.

B

Bachelor—*Dokushin* (Doke-sheen).
Also, *hitorimono* (he-toe-ree-moe-no), and the old word,
chonga (chone-gah).

I am still a bachelor.
Boku wa mada dokushin desu
(Boe-kuu wah mah-dah doke-sheen dess).

Bar—*Ba* (Baah).
This is a "regular" Western-style bar or lounge. Bars that are more traditionally Japanese in decor and style are known as *sakaba* (sah-kah-baah). One's favorite bar is known as *yukitsuke-no ba* (yuu-keet'sue-kay-no baah).

Balls, testicles—*Kogan* (Koe-ghan).
This is the medical term for the male testes. In everyday parlance, the gonads are often referred to as *kin tama* (keen tah-mah) or "golden balls," indicative of the value with which they were once regarded. Other old terms include *tama tama* (tah-mah tah-mah), literally "ball ball" or two balls; and *ke-no tama* (kay-no tah-mah), or "balls with hair."

Bath—*Ofuro* (Oh-fuu-roe).
Bathing in scorching hot water is an ancient Japanese custom. The sexes bathed together, most in large public baths, until the early 1950s when it was prohibited in public commercial baths as being "uncivilized"—primarily as a result of Christian-oriented female members of the Diet.

Family bath—*Kazoku buro* (Kah-zoe-kuu buu-roe).
Bath-for-two – *Fufu buro* (Fuu-fuu buu-roe). Many inns and hot spring resort hotels have double-sized baths especially designed to accommodate two persons. *Fufu* means husband and wife, but in such places couples do not have to produce a marriage license to bathe together. Some resort inns have baths big enough to accommodate several dozen people at the same time. Mixed-bathing is called *Konyoku-buro* (Kone-yoe-kuu-buu-roe).

Beautiful—*Utsukushii* (Ut-sue-kuu-shee).

You are beautiful.
Anata wa utsukushii desu.
(Ah-nah-tah wah ut-sue-kuu-shee dess).

That is a beautiful dress.
Sore wa utsukushii doresu desu.
(Soe-ray wah ut-sue-kuu-shee doeray-sue dess).

Beauty—*Utsukushisa* (Ut-sue-kuu-she-sah).

Her beauty is extraordinary.
Kanojo no utsukushisa wa taishita mono desu.
(Kah-no-joe no ut-sue-kuu-she-sah wa tie-ssh-tah
moe-no dess).

In compound words and sayings, *bi* (bee), also means beauty.

Beauty is only skin deep (a proverb).
Bi mo kawa hitoe.
(Bee moe kah-wah ssh-toe-eh).

Beautiful girl—*Bijin* (Bee-jeen).
Also, *utsukushii onna* (Ut-sue-kuu-shee own-nah).

There are many beautiful women in the northern area of
Honshu.
Honshu no kita-no ho ni bijin ga takusan imasu.
(Hone-shuu no kee-tah-no hoe nee bee-jeen gah tock-sahn
ee-mahss).

Bed—*Bedo* (Bay-doe).
Also, **betto** (bet-toe).
The Japanese word for this very popular piece of furniture is *shindai* (sheen-die). Many Japanese now sleep on beds instead of the traditional *futon* (fuu-tone) floor mattresses.

Beer—*Biiru* (Bee-rue).
Bottled beer—*Bin biiru* (Bean bee-rue); **large bottle**—*obin* (ohh-bean); **small bottle**—*kobin* (koe-bean); **draft beer**—*nama biiru* (nah-mah bee-rue); **dark or black beer**—*kuro biiru* (kuu-roe bee-rue). **Beer hall**—*Biya horu* (bee-yah hoe-rue).

Beer, please.
Biiru wo kudasai
(Bee-rue oh kuu-dah-sie).

Beginner—*Shinmai* (Sheen-my).
A young man or woman just learning how to make love may be described as *shinmai*.

Big—*Okii* (Ohh-kee).
Big eyes are regarded as especially attractive among the Japanese.

Your eyes are really large, aren't they!
Anata-no me wa okii desu, ne!
(Ah-nah-tah-no may wah ooh-kee dess, nay!)

Birth control—*Sanji seigen* (Sahn-jee say-e-gain).
Also, *hinin* (he-neen).

Do you practice birth control?
Anata wa sanji seigen wo shite imasu ka?
(Ah-nah-tah wah sahn-jee say-e-gain oh ssh-tay
ee-mahss kah?)

Birthday—*Tanjobi* (Tahn-joe-be).

When is your birthday?
Anata no tanjobi wa itsu desu ka?
(Ah-nah-tah no tahn-joe-be wah eet-sue dess kah?)

My birthday is tomorrow.
Watakushi no tanjobi wa ashita desu.
(Wah-tock-she no tahn-joe-be wah ah-sshtah dess.)

Blue day—*Seiri bi* (Say-e-ree bee).
The day, or days, when a woman is in her menstrual period.
Perhaps even more common is *hata bi* (hah-tah bee) or "flag
day," which is also Japan's "flag day" from the fact that the
national flag is a red dot on a white background. *Hata Bi* is
a national holiday in Japan, thus a double reference to a
woman's monthly period.

Blush—*Sekimen* (Say-kee-mane).

Why are you blushing?
Doshite sekimen shite imasu ka?
(Doe-ssh-tay say-kee-mane ssh-tay ee-mahss kah?)

Body—*Karada* (Kah-rah-dah).

She likes men with big bodies.
Kanojo wa karada no okii otoko ga suki desu.
(Kahno-joe wah kah-rah-dah no ohh-kee oh-toe-koe
gah ski des).

Boy-crazy—*Otoko-kichigai* (Oh-toe-koe-kee-chee-guy).

Your girlfriend is boy-crazy!
Anata no garu furendo wa otoko-kichigai desu.
(Ah-nah-tah no gah-rue fuu-rendoe wah oh-toe-koe kee-
chee-guy dess).

Boyfriend—*Kareshi* (Kah-ray-she).
Also, and much more common, *boifurendo* (boy fuu-ren-
doe).

Do you have a boyfriend?
Boifurendo ga imasu ka?
(Boy fuu-ren-doe gah ee-mahss kah?)

Bra—*Bura* (Buu-rah).
Brassiere—*Burajrya* (Buu-rah-jee-yah). The wearing of bras
did not become common in Japan until the late 1950s. Some
women still do not wear them. *No bura* (from the English)
was once a popular term among young braless girls.

Break up—*Wakareru* (Wah-kah-ray-rue).
Also, *en wo kiru* (inn oh kee-rue).

Are you going to break up with him?
Anata wa kare to wakaremasu ka?
(Ah-nah-tah wah kah-ray toe wah-kah-ray-mahss kah?)

Let's break up.
En wo kirimasho
(Inn oh kee-ree-mah-show).

Bride—*Hanayome* (Hah-nah-yoe-may).
In Japanese *hanayome* is written in ideograms meaning
"flower, woman, house"—the idea being that a woman as
pretty and as fresh as a flower goes to another house when
she marries.

Bridegroom—*Hanamuko* (Hah-nah-muu-koe).
The etymology of this word throws most Japanese. It is written
with characters that mean "flower, woman, help"—which
could be construed to mean something like "helping a flower-
like woman."

Breasts—*Chichi* (Chee-chee).
Also, *oppai* (ope-pie). **Nipples**—*Chibusa* (Chee-buu-sah).

Let me see your breasts.
Oppai wo misete kudasai
(Ope-pie oh me-say-tay kuu-dah-sie)

Broke (moneyless)—*Okane ga nai* (Oh-kah-nay gah nie).
A more vulgar form is *kara-ketsu* (kah-rah-kate-sue) or "empty ass."

> I am broke. (Or, My ass is empty!)
> *Boku wa kara-ketsu da!*
> (Boe-kuu wah kah-rah kate-sue dah!)

Bust (female breasts)—*Basuto* (Bah-sue-toe).
In earlier years in Japan female breasts were not sex objects. In fact, they were de-emphasized and flattened as much as possible. Big breasts were therefore considered more of a handicap than an asset. This attitude has changed—and Japanese breasts are getting larger as a result of changes in the diet.

C

Cabaret—*Kyabare* (K'yah-bah-ray).
The terms cabaret, nightclub, lounge, and hostess bar or hostess lounge are used more or less interchangeably in Japan, but under the law if a place employs hostesses it is legally listed as a cabaret. In "true" cabarets, hostesses are automatically assigned to each customer or group of customers when they come in. Hostess bars and hostess lounges also generally follow this practice. In so-called nightclubs, which are operated more or less foreign-style, customers sometimes have the option of requesting hostesses or drinking alone.

Regular patrons in cabarets often request specific girls in a custom known as *go-shimei* (go-she-may). When they do, there is an extra charge. On other occasions, hostesses are assigned by the cabaret, following a pre-arranged order.

It is also the custom for cabarets to rotate the hostesses every twenty or thirty minutes, usually sending in new girls one at a time. Each time a new girl joins a party she is added to the customer's bill. Foreigners who wander into cabarets and are not familiar with this system are often shocked at being charged for several hostesses they "didn't order."

Call girl—*Koru garu* (Koe-rue gah-rue).
There are numerous call-girl rings operating in Japan under different guises. One of the most common ploys is private guides for shopping or touring.

Car—*Jidosha* (Jee-doe-shah).
Also, *kuruma* (kuu-rue-mah).

Let's go by car.
Jidosha de ikimasho.
(Jee-doe-shah day ee-kee-mah-show).

Car sex—*Ka sekusu* (Kah sake-sue).
This refers, of course, to having sex in a car—a common practice among the young.

Can you lay the seat back?
Shiito wo sageru koto ga dekimasu ka?
(Shee-toe oh sah-gay-rue koe-toe gah day-kee-mahss kah?)

Caress, fondle—*Aibu-suru* (Aye-buu-sue-rue).

He is always caressing his girlfriend.
Kare wa garufurendo wo itsumo aibu-shite imasu.
(Kah-ray wah gah-rue-fuu-ren-doe oh eet-sue-moe aye-buu-
ssh-tay ee-mahss).

Cartoons for adults—*Otona-no manga* (Oh-toe-nah-no
mahn-gah).
Adult cartoons are cartoon comics with explicitly illustrated
sexual themes—the most common form of pornography in
Japan.

Do you read adult comics?
Otona-no manga wo yomimasu ka?
(Oh-toe-nah-no mahn-gah oh yoe-me-mahss kah?)

Chastity—*Teiso* (Tay-e-soe). **Chastity belt**—*Teiso tai* (Tay-
e-soe tie).

Is your boyfriend faithful to you?
Anata-no boifurendo wa teiso-no tadashii hito desu ka?
(Ah-nah-tah-no boy fuu-ren-doe wah tay-e-soe-no tah-dah-
shee ssh-toe dess kah?)

He is trying to seduce that girl ("break her chastity").
Kare wa ano onna-no-ko no teiso wo
yaburo to shite imasu.
(Kah-ray wah ah-no own-nah-no-koe no tay-e-soe oh
yah-buu-roh toe ssh-tay ee-mahss.)

Charming—*Miryoku ga aru* (Mee-rio-kuu gah ah-rue).
Also, *aikyo ga aru* (aye-k'yoe gah ah-rue).

She is a charming woman.
Kanojo wa miryoku ga aru onna-no-hito desu.
(Kah-no-joe wah mee-rio-kuu gah ah-rue own-nah-no-ssh-
toe dess).

Checkup for VD—*Baidoku kensa* (By-doe-kuu kane-sah).

Please examine me for venereal disease.
Baidoku kensa wo shite kudasai.
(By-doe-kuu kane-sah oh ssh-tay kuu-dah-sie)

Cherry boy—*Cheri boi* (Chay-ree boy).
So many of the young American GIs who took part in the
military Occupation of Japan had had no sexual experience
that the term "cherry boy" was one of the first "new words"
the GIs learned. Japanese prostitutes delighted at breaking in
"cherry boys" and would often service them without large
fees (resulting in some GIs faking virginity over and over
again). *Cherry girl* was also used. The Japanese word for a
male virgin is *dotei* (doe-tay). A virgin girl is a *shojo* (show-
joe).

Clap—*Rimbyo* (Reem-b'yoe).
Also, *rin-chan* (reen-chan), which is a diminutive form that
might be translated as "clappy." Whatever the word, it is
gonorrhea.

Be careful of clap.

Rimbyo wo ki wo tsuke-nasai.

(Reem-b'yoe oh kee oh t'skay-nah-sie.)

Climax, sexual—*Shasei suru* (Shah-say-e sue-rue).

This is the "technical" term. The word most people use is quite different. In the Japanese lexicon of love, you do not "come." You "go." Or, *iku* (ee-kuu).

When foreigners first learn this interesting difference, they are sometimes so confused they don't know whether to "come" or "go."

I'm coming! I'm coming!

Iku! Iku!

(Ee-kuu! Ee-kuu!)

I'm going to go!

Itchao!

(Ee-chah-oh!)

I went.

Itchatta.

(Ee-chah-tah.)

Clitoris—*Inkaku* (Inn-kah-kuu).

This is the medical term. Vulgar terms include *saneko* (sah-nay-koe) and *osane* (oh-sah-nay).

Cock-teaser—*Jirashiya* (Jee-rah-she-yah).
Also, *hi kakeya* (he kah-kay-yah), or "one who lights fire."
Another old term: *hi-ga kashi* (he-gah kah-she).

That broad is just a cock-teaser.
Ano suke wa jirashiya dake desu
(Ah-no skay wah jee-rah-she-yah dah-kay dess).

Cold-blooded man—*Tsumetai otoko* (T'sue-may-tie oh-toe koe).
Cold-blooded woman—*Tsumetai onna* (T'sue-may-tie own-nah).

He is cold-blooded so women do not like him.
Kare wa tsumetai otoko dakara onna ni sukare nai.
(Kah-ray wah t'sue-may-tie oh-toe-koe dah-kah-rah own-
nah nee sue-kah-re nah-ee).

Consolation money—*Isha ryo* (Ee-shah rio).
In Japan when men break up with mistresses or wives, they
often have to pay large sums of "consolation money."

How much consolation money did he pay?
Kare wa isharyo wo ikura haraimashita ka?
(Kah-ray wah ee-shah rio oh ee-kuu-rah hah-rye-mahssh-
tah kah?)

Contraceptive—*Hiningu* (He-neen-guu).

Are you using a contraceptive?
Anata wa hiningu wo tsukatte imasu ka?
(An-nah-tah wah he-neen-guu oh scot-tay ee-mahss kah?)

Copulate—*Seiko suru* (Say-ee-koe sue-rue).
There are several terms used in reference to sexual intercourse.
The most common is *neru* (nay-rue) or "sleep" as in "sleep
with." A more vulgar term that has the connotation of "screw"
is *yaru* (yah-rue), literally "to do."

Common-law marriage—*Nai-en* (Nie-inn).
Common-law husband—*Nai-en no otto* (Nie-inn no oat-
toe). **Common-law wife**—*Nai-en no tsuma* (Nie-inn no t'sue-
mah).

She is his common-law wife.
Kanojo wa kare no naien no tsuma desu.
(Kah-no-joe wah kah-ray no nie-inn no t'sue-mah dess)

Country girl—*Inaka-no ko* (Ee-nah-kah-no koe)
Girls fresh in from the country are notorious in Japan for being
naive and easily deceived by unscrupulous men. Because of
this they are frequently sought after as attendants in massage
parlors and employees in other sex-oriented type businesses.

Country hick—*Inakappei* (Ee-nah-kah-pay).
Young men and women just in from the outlying provinces who are not familiar with big city ways are often called *inakappei*, generally in a friendly or humorous way.

Court, woo—*Iiyoru* (Ee-yoe-rue). Also, *yuwaku* (yuu-wah-kuu).

Are you courting that woman?
Anata wa ano onna-no-hito ni iiyotte imasu ka?
(Ah-nah-tah wah ah-no own-nah-no-ssh-toe ni ee-yoe-tay ee-mahss kah?)

Cry—*Naku* (Nah-kuu).
Cry baby—*Naki mushi* (Nah-kee muu-she). **Crocodile tears**—*Uso naki* (Uu-so nah-kee). **"Deceiving tears"**—*Damashi naki* (Dah-mah-she nah-kee). Japanese girls cry easily and often use tears to influence men.

Don't cry!
Nakanai de!
(Nah-kah-nie day!)

Why are you crying?
Doshite naite imasu ka?
(Doh-ssh-tay nie-tay ee-mahss kah?)

Cunnilingus—*Name-name suru* (Nah-may-nah-may sue-rue). This is from the word *nameru* (nah-may-rue), meaning "to lick." There are several other words to express the same idea, such as *ai-name* (aye-nah-may), when a man and a woman perform oral sex on each other. The literal translation is "love-lick."

Customer—*Okyaku-san* (Oh-kyack-sahn).
In Japan the word for guest and customer is the same, and is indicative of the kind of service and attention generally given to customers and guests. Someone who is a regular client of a shop, bar, brothel, or soapland is ofren called *Otokui-san* (Oh-toe-kuu-e-sahn) or "Mr. Preferred Customer," and given special consideration. When business establishments do not know a customer's name, they will address him or her as *Okyaku-san*.

Cute—*Kawaii* (Kah-wah-ee).
Young Japanese girls (and small things) are often especially cute, and this word gets a lot of use.

Isn't she (it) cute!
Kawaii desu ne!
(Kah-wah-ee dess, nay!)

Japanese women who are in the sex business will often tell a man his penis is *kawaii* if it is smaller than average or smaller than they expected. It is *not* a compliment.

D

Daisy chain—*Toripuru purei* (Toe-reep-puu-rue pue-ray-e). This is from the English "triple play," and refers to several people engaging in group sex. In soapland argot, two girls servicing one man is known as *ni-rinsha* (nee-reen-shah) or a two-wheeled vehicle (bicycle). Three girls and one man is a *san-rinsha* (sahn-reen-shah) or three-wheeler (tricycle).

Dance—*Odoru* (Oh-doe-rue).

Let's dance!
Odorimasho!
(Oh-doe-ree-mah-show!)

Would you like to dance?
Odori wa ikaga desu ka?
(Oh-doe-ree wah ee-kah-gah dess kah?)

Date—*Deito* (Day-e-toe).

How about a date tonight?
Komban deito shimasen ka?
(Kome-bahn day-e-toe she-mah-sin kah?)

What time must you be in (from a date)?*
Mongen wa nanji desu ka?
(Moan-gain wah nahn-jee dess kah?)

*The original meaning of this old term refers to gate or door closing time.

Daughter—*Musume* (Muu-sue-may).
An old word used in reference to the daughters of the rich is *reijo* (ray-e-joe). Daughters of the wealthy tend to have the reputation of being playgirls.

Dear—*Anata* (Ah-nah-tah).
This word literally means "you," but when used by itself (commonly by women and only rarely by men), it is the equivalent of the English term, "dear"—as in, "Dear, that isn't the way it's done." It is not used as a form of written address, as in "Dear Mrs. Jones."

Dictionary with arms and legs—*Te-ashi no tsuita jibiki* (Tay-ah-she no t'sue-ee-tah jee-bee-kee).
A "dictionary with arms and legs" is sometimes used in reference to a young woman living with a foreign student who is studying Japanese. "Living dictionary" or *iki jibiki* (ee-kee jee-bee-kee) is also sometimes used in reference to the Japanese girlfriend of a foreign student.

Dildo—*Harigata* (Hah-ree-gah-tah).
Dildoes, some in the shape of gods, have long been popular in Japan. Vibrating dildoes and other sexual accessories are now popularly called *otona no omocha* (oh-toe-nah no oh-moe-chah) or "adult toys," and are sold in adult toy shops. Present-day dildoes go up and down and move in a circle. These adult toy shops are also known as *poruno shoppu* (poe-rue-no shope-puu).

Doll—*Ningyo* (Neen-g'yoe).
Young Japanese girls are often compared to dolls in both size and beauty.

> You are like a doll.
> *Anata wa ningyo no yoh desu.*
> (Ah-nah-tah wah neen-g'yoe no yohh dess).

Double-cross—*Uragiru* (Uu-rah-ghee-rue).

> I was double-crossed by my girlfriend.
> *Boku wa garu furendo ni uragirareta.*
> (Boe-kuu wah gah-rue fuu-ren-doe ni
> uu-rah-ghee-rah-ray-tah).

Down there—*Shita* (Ssh-tah).
"Down there" is a euphemism for the genital organs. So is *are* (ah-ray), meaning "that."

Drag show—*Homo sho* (Hoe-moe show).
Also, *Okama sho* (Oh-kah-mah show), and *reza* (ray-zah) show. A number of nightclubs in Tokyo feature homosexual lesbian shows.

> I saw a very interesting homosexual show last night.
> *Yube taihen omoshiroi homo sho wo mimashita.*
> (Yuu-bay tie-hane oh-moe-shee-roy hoe-moe show oh me-
> mah-ssh-tah).

Drink—*Nomu* (No-muu).

A drinking buddy is called a *nomi nakama* (No-me nah-kah-mah). Drinking money is *nomi shiro* (no-me she-roe). Drinking place is *nomi ya* (no-me yah).

Let's go drinking.
Nomi ni ikimasho.
(No-me nee ee-kee-mah-show)

There are many types of drinking places in Japan. *Nomi ya* is a generic term generally referring to a neighborhood-type bar or stand-up-bar patronized by lower class laborers. Such bars abound in the vicinity of commuter train and subway stations.

Drunk—*Yopparai* (Yope-pah-rye). **Drunkard**—*Nombe* (Nome-bay).

He gets drunk every night.
Anohito wa maiban yopparatte imasu.
(Ah-no-ssh-toe wah my-bahn yope-pah-rot-tay ee-mahss).

He is a drunkard.
Kare wah nombe desu
(Kah-ray wah nome-bay dess).

E

Engagement—*Konyaku* (Kone-yah-kuu).
To become engaged—*Konyaku suru* (Kone-yah-kuu sue-rue).

Are you engaged to him?
Anata wa anohito to konyaku shite imasu ka?
(Ah-nah-tah wah ah-no-ssh-toe toe kone-yah-kuu ssh-tay
ee-mahss kah?)

Engagement ring—*Engeji ringu* (En-gay-jee reen-guu).
Both the concept and the words were adopted from America
in the 1960s.

Is that an engagement ring?
Sore wa engeji ringu desu ka?
(Soe-ray wah en-gay-jee reen-guu dess kah?)

Enjoy—*Tanoshimimasu* (Tah-no-she-me-mahss).

Are you enjoying yourself?
Tanoshinde imasu ka?
(Tah-no-sheen-day ee-mahss-kah?)

Entice—*Sosonokasu* (Soe-soe-no-kah-sue).

He enticed her into working as a soapland girl.
*Kare wa kanojo ni sopurando de hataraku yo ni
sosonokashi mashita.*
(Kah-ray wah kah-no-joe nee soe-puu-rahn-doe day hah-
tah-rah-kuu yoe nee soe-soe-no-kah-she mahss-tah.)

Erection—*Bokii* (Boe-kee-e).

To get an erection—*Chimbo ga katakunaru* (Cheem-boe gah kah-tah-kuu-nah-rue). *Katakunaru* means "to get hard." Also: *chimbo ga tatsu* (Cheem-boe gah tot-sue), or "the penis stands up."

> My goodness! Your penis is standing up!
> *Ara! Anata-no chimbo ga tatte imasu!*
> (Ah-rah! Ah-nah-tah-no cheem-boe gah tot-tay ee-mahss!)

Another term used in reference to the erection of the male phallus is *okosu* (oh-koe-sue), which means "to wake up," or "rise up." Another one: *okiku naru* (oh-kee-kuu nah-rue)— "to get big."

Extra-marital sex—*Uwaki wo suru* (Uu-wah-kee oh sue-rue).

Most foreign men in Japan are frequently asked if they engage in extra-marital sex.

> Do you engage in extra-marital sex?
> *Anata wa uwaki wo shimasu ka?*
> (Ah-nah-tah wah uuu-wah-kee oh she-mahss kah?).

Extend time—*Jikan wo encho suru* (Jee-khan oh en-choe sue-rue).

In soaplands and similar situations, when a customer is having fun with a girl and wants to go beyond the normal one hour, he may extend the period of time in thirty-minute and one-hour increments.

Please extend my time.
Jikan wo encho shite kudasai
(Jee-khan oh en-choe ssh-tay kuu-dah-sie.)

F

Fall in love—*Koi ni ochiru* (Koy nee oh-chee-rue).
Also, *aishimashita* (aye-she-mahssh-tah); and *horeru* (hoe-ray-rue). To be in love is called *renai no naka* (rain-aye no nah-kah).

I fell in love last night.
Yube watakushi wa koi ni ochimashita
(Yuu-bay wah-tock-she wah koy nee oh-chee-mahssh-tah).

I have fallen in love with you.
Watakushi wa anata ni horeta.
(Wah-tock-she wah ah-nah-tah nee hoe-rate-tah)

Are you in love with her?
Anata wa kanojo to renai no naka desu ka?
(Ah-nah-tah wah kah-no-joe toe rain-aye no nah-kah
dess kah?)

"Fast shooter"—*Haya uchi* (Hah-yah uu-chee).
This is the equivalent of "fast-on-the-draw" as well as "quick-comer"—the latter referring to a man who has a sexual climax quickly, usually too fast for his partner's satisfaction. Another expression used to describe the fast climaxer is *san-koki-han*

(sahn-koe-kee-hahn), literally "three-and-a-half strokes." In other words, a man who "goes" after three and a half strokes.

Fat—*Futotte iru* (Fuu-tote-tay ee-rue).
Fatso—*Debu-chan* (Day-buu-chahn).

> You've put on weight, haven't you!
> *Futorimashita, ne!*
> (Fuu-toe-ree-mahssh-tah, nay!)

> She is too fat.
> *Kanojo wa futori sugimasu*
> (Kah-no-joe wah fuu-toe-ree sue-ghee-mahss).

Fellatio—*Ferachio* (Fay-rah-chee-oh).
Also, *shakuhachi* (shah-kuu-hah-chee). The former is, of course, the Japanization of the English word. The latter actually means "flute" but is commonly used in reference to a woman performing oral sex on a man. Another derivative of the English word that developed in the soaplands is *ofera* (oh-fay-rah). *Deepu Suroto* (Dee-puu Sue-roe-toe) from the movie "Deep Throat" was in vogue for a while.

Female—*Josei* (Joe-say-e).
This literally means "female sex." The word for woman is *onna* (own-nah).

Female on top—*Chausu* (Chah-ou-sue).
This is one of the positions on the famous "sex position charts" that used to be given to newlyweds on their wedding night.

Fiancé—*Konyaku-no otoko* (Kone-yah-kuu-no oh-toe-koe).
Also, *konyaku-sha* (kone-yah-kuu-shah).

This is my fiancé.
Kono kata wa watakushi no konyakusha desu.
(Koe-no kah-tah wah wah-tock-she no
kone-yah-kuu-shah dess).

Fiancee—*Konyakuchu-no onna* (Kone-yah-kuu-chuu-no own-nah).
Also, *konyakusha* (kone-yah-kuu-shah).

First love—*Hatsu-koi* (Hot-sue-koy).
Japanese, especially young girls, romanticize the concept and practice of first love.

She was my first love.
Kanojo wa watakushi no hatsu-koi deshita.
(Kah-no-joe wah wah-tock-she no hot-sue-koy desh-tah)

Flattery—*Oseji* (Oh-say-jee).
Flattery is a polished art in Japan.

I don't need your flattery!
Oseji wa iranai!
(Oh-say-jee wah ee-rah-nie!)

Flip for—*Noboseru* (No-boe-say-rue).
Also, *muchu ni naru* (muu-chuu nee nah-rue).

She really flipped for that guy.
Kanojo wa ano otoko ni honki de muchu ni narimashita
(Kah-no-joe wah ah-no oh-toe-koe nee hoan-kee day muu-
chuu nee nah-ree-mah-ssh-tah).

Flirt—*Ichatsuku* (Ee-chah-t'sue-kuu).
Also: *icha-icha suru* (ee-chah-ee-chah sue-rue); *beta-beta
suru* (bay-tah bay-tah sue-rue); *jareru* (jah-ray-rue).

You'd better stop flirting with that guy! (said by a girl)
Ano otoko to icha-icha shinai ho ga iin da wa!
(Ah-no oh-toe-koe toe ee-chah-ee-chah she-nie hoh gah een
dah wah!)

"Floating World"—*Ukiyo* (Uu-kee-yoe).
The Japanese traditionally regarded life as fragile and
transitory, particularly in its more pleasurable aspects. Thus,
the so-called entertainment trades (drinking places, sporting
places, etc.) have long been associated with the literary allusion
of *ukiyo* or "the world that is floating."

Foreigner—*Gaijin* (Guy-jeen).
To the Japanese, anyone who is not both racially and ethnically
Japanese is a *gaijin*, or "outside person." **Foreign man**—
Gaijin-no otoko (Guy-jeen-no oh-toe-koe); **foreign woman**
—*gaijin-no onna* (guy-jeen-no own-nah).

Foxy—*Ikasu* (Eee-kah-sue).

She is a very foxy (sexually attractive, charming, etc.)
lady.
Kanojo wa taihen ikasu josei desu.
(Kah-no-joe wah tie-hane ee-kah-suu joe-saye dess.)

Free sex – *Furii sekusu* (Fuu-ree say-kuu'sue).
In the 1970s small groups of avant-garde young Japanese
women began practicing "free sex" as a protest against the
growing materialism of society.

Are you against free sex?
Anata wa furii sekusu ni hantai desu ka?
(Ah-nah-tah wah fuu-ree say-kuu'sue ni hahn-tie dess kah?)

French kiss – *Furenchi kisu* (Fuu-rane-chee kee-sue).
Unsophisticated girls who do not recognize this term usually
get the idea when it is demonstrated to them.

Quick, give me a French kiss!
Hayaku, Furenchi kisu kure, yo!
(Hah-yah-kuu, Fuu-rane-chee kee-sue kuu-ray, yoe!)

Fuck – *Seiko suru* (Say-e-koe sue-rue). This is the equivalent
of "sexual intercourse." The vulgar "four letter" version is
omanko wo yaru (oh-mahn-koe oh yah-rue). Younger Japanese
and many of those who have had sexual experiences in the
United States or elsewhere as students or tourists often use
faku (fah-kuu).

G

Gang-bang—*Mawashi* (Mah-wah-she).
This word comes from *mawasu* (mah-wah-sue), meaning "to revolve, spin, pass around." To be understood in the sexual sense it must be used in the right context.

Gang-rape—*Rinkan sareru* (reen-khan sah-ray-rue).

Those two sisters were gang-raped.
Sono kyodai no onnano-ko wa rinkan saremashita.
(Soe-no k'yoe-die no own-nah-no-koe wa reen-khan sah-ray-mahssh-tah).

Gay bar—*Gei ba* (Gay-e baah).
Japan's major cities generally have a number of well-known gay bars.

He wants to go to a gay bar.
Kare wa gei ba ni ikitai desu
(Kah-ray wah gay-e baah nee ee-kee-tie dess.)

Gay man—*Onna girai* (Own-nah ghee-rye).
Japan has a history of bisexual love, particularly between men and boys, so homosexuality has never been the object of as much scorn or criticism as it has in some Western countries. *Onna girai* literally means someone who dislikes women, "woman hater."

He is gay (homosexual).
Anohito wa onna girai desu
(Ah-no-ssh-toe wah own-nah ghee-rye dess)

Gay woman—*Otoko girai* (Oh-toe-koe ghee-rye).
Also, *rezu* (ray-zuu). Since Japanese men traditionally had almost unlimited access to casual sexual relationships before and after marriage, lesbian relationships among girls and women were relatively common in early Japan. Now they are no more common than elsewhere.

Gentleman—*Shinshi* (Sheen-she).
Also, *gentoruman* (gen-toe-rue-mahn).

He is really a gentleman.
Anohito wa honto ni shinshi desu.
(Ah-no-ssh-toe wah hoan-toe nee sheen-she dess.)

Get sexually excited—*Kofun suru* (Koe-hune sue-rue).

When an attractive woman touches me I get sexually excited.
Miryokuteki na onna ga boku ni sawaru to kofun shimasu.
(Mee-rio-kuu-tay-kee nah own-nah gah boekuu nee sah-wah-rue toe koe-hune she-mahss).

Geisha—*Geisha* (Gay-e-shah).
A "person skilled in the art of entertainment," geisha are still an important part of Japan's "floating world." High-level politicians in particular patronize geisha as a tradition.

Girl—*Onna-no-ko* (Own-nah-no-koe).
This word is often used interchangeably with *ojo-san*, in reference to unmarried women.

> What a pretty girl! (male speech)
> *Kirei na onna-no-ko da, ne!*
> (Kee-ray na own-nah-no-koe dah, nay!)

> Do you know that girl?
> *Ano onna-no-ko wo shitte imasu ka?*
> (Ah-no own-nah-no-koe oh ssh-tay ee-mahss kah?)

Girlfriend—*Garu furendo* (Gah-rue fuu-ren-doe).
Also, *kanojo* (kah-no-joe).

> This is Suzuki's girlfriend.
> *Konohito wa Suzuki-san no garu furendo desu.*
> (Koe-no-ssh-toe wah Suu-zoo-kee-sahn no gah-rue fuu-ren-doe dess.)

My girl (in vulgar slang): *Ore no suke* (Oh-ray no skay).

Girl clever at fooling men—*Zurugashikoi onna* (Zuu-rue-gah-she-koy own-nah).
Many of the women in Japan's huge pleasure trades become especially clever at leading men on and manipulating them for their own ends.

That woman is especially clever (in handling men).
Sono onna wa toku ni zurngashikoi desu.
(Soe-no own-nah wa toe-kuu nee zuu-rue-gah-she-koy
dess.)

Girl-crazy—*Onna-kichigai* (Own-nah kee-chee-guy).

Many young men are girl-crazy.
Takusan no wakai otoko-no-hito wa onna-kichigai desu.
(Tock-sahn no wah-kie oh-toe-koe-no-ssh-toe wah own-nah
kee-chee-guy dess.)

I am crazy about you.
Boku wa anata ni muchu desu.
(Boe-kuu wah ah-nah-tah nee muu-chuu dess.)

Girl especially attractive to men—*Moteru onna* (Moe-tay-
rue own-nah).

Who is the most sought-after hostess in the club?
Kurabu de ichiban moteru onna wa donata desu ka?
(Kuu-rah-buu day ee-chee-bahn moetay-rue own-nah wah
doe-nah-tah dess kah?)

Girl Hunt—*Garu hanto* (gah-rue hahn-goe).
Japanese men often visit coffee shops, bars, marinas, and
musical events looking for girls to pick up. Girls also go on
boi hanto (boy hahn-toe).

Gonorrhea—*Rimbyo* (Reem-b'yoe).
This literally means "the lonely disease," which is pretty graphic. Gonorrhea is one of the most common sexually transmitted diseases in Japan. The major venereal diseases were unknown in Japan until brought there by Portugese sailors in 1543, when they were shipwrecked on Tanega Island south of Kyushu.

Goodbye—*Sayonara* (Sah-yoe-nah-rah).
This word is as beautiful as Hawaii's provocative "aloha." It means "If it must be so" (we will part).

I cannot say goodbye to you.
Anata ni sayonara to doshite mo iemasen!
(Ah-nah-tah nee sah-yoe-nah-rah toe dosh-tay moe ee-eh-mah-sin).

Good style—*Sutairu ga ii* (Sue-tie-rue gah ee).
This generally refers to a person with a good figure-slender, shapely, and fairly tall. It is perhaps more often used to describe men than women.

Good wife—*Ii oku-san* (Ee-oak-sahn).
In earlier years an *ii oku-san* was one who did not complain, regardless of her husband's behavior at home or his outside peccadilloes. The term is still heard, but more likely when a Japanese male is describing Japanese wives in general.

Isn't she (aren't you) a good wife!
Ii oku-san da, ne!
(Ee oak-sahn dah, nay!)

Going with a girl/woman—*Onna to tsukiau* (Own-nah toe t'sue-kee-ow).

Is he going with that woman?
Kare wa ana onna to tsukiatte imasu ka?
(Kah-ray wah ah-no own-nah toe t'sue-kee-aht-tay
ee-mahss kah?)

Greatest—*Saiko* (Sie-koe).
This word is often used to describe an unusually attractive person or an extraordinarily pleasurable experience.

She is the greatest!
Kanojo wa saiko desu!
(Kah-no-joe wah sie-koe dess.)

Gross man—*Kimochi warui otoko* (Kee-moe-chee wah-rue-e oh-toe-koe).
This expression is usually used by Japanese women to describe men who really turn them off. They will sometimes make a point of using it to put a foreign man down when they want to impress Jaapanese men with their Japaneseness. A *kimochi warui otoko* makes them "feel bad."

Groupie—*Shineitai* (Sheen-eh-ee-tie).
Originally this term applied to military-type bodyguards, and later came to be used in reference to prostitutes who followed and serviced troops in the field. Now it means the girls and women who vie to have sex with popular entertainers.

H

Hair—*Kami-no-ke* (Kah-me-no-kay).
Figuratively this is "head hair." In context, just *kami* will do.

Your hair is pretty.
Anata no kami wa kirei desu.
(Ah-nah-tah no kah-me wah kee-ray dess.)

Hair-of-the-dog—*Mukae-zake* (Muu-kie zah-kay).
Mukae means "to meet," and *zake* is sake, with the reference being the drink that meets you on the way from a hangover.

Hair-on-chest—*Mune-ge* (Muu-nay-gay).
The Japanese equate hair on the chest—rare among Japanese men—with extraordinary manliness (verging on the animalistic). Japanese girls typically make a fuss over men with lots of chest hair, and like to run their fingers through it.

Hairy—*Keppoi* (Kape-poy).
Also, *kebukai* (kay-buu-kie). Japanese women are fascinated—but also a little frightened—by men who are very hairy. Hairiness is usually associated with both masculinity and beastliness.

Hairy barbarian—*Ketto yabanjin* (Kate-toe yah-bahn-jeen).
To the highly refined, clean, and carefully groomed Japanese
of the 16th and 17th centuries, the bearded and usually dirty
Westerners they first came into contact with had the
appearance and often the manners of *ketto yabanjin*. The
phrase is still used occasionally in a highly derogatory sense.

Handsome man—*Ii otoko* (Ee oh-toe-koe).
Japanese women often say they do not like handsome men
"because they cannot be trusted." They fall for them
nevertheless.

Isn't he a handsome man!
Ma! Anohito wa ii otoko desu, ne!
(Mah! Ah-no-ssh-toe wah ee oh-toe-koe dess, nay!)

Hangover—*Futsuka yoi* (Futes-kah yoy).
Futsuka (Futes-kah) means "two days" and *yoi* (yoy) means
to "stagger"—i.e., something that makes you wobbly for two
days.

I have a hangover.
Futsuka yoi shite imasu.
(Futes-kah yoy ssh-tay ee-mahss.)

Happy—*Ureshii* (Uu-ray-she).
This word expresses happiness of the moment. *Shiawase* (she-
ah-wah-say) is happiness that lasts for a little longer period;
and *kofuku* (koe-fuu-kuu) for a still longer time. A state of
continuous happiness is expressed by *tanoshimimasu* (tah-no-
she-mee-mahss).

Thanks to you, I am very happy.
Anata no okage de watakushi wa taihen kofuku desu.
(An-nah-tah no oh-kah-gay day wah-tock-she wah tie-hane
koe-fuu-kuu dess.)

I am happy with my life.
Watakushi no seikatsu wa totemo tanoshii desu.
(Wah-tock-she no say-kot-sue wah toe-tay-moe
tah-no-she-e dess.)

Hate—*Kirai* (Kee-rye).
"Big hate"—*Dai kirai* (Die kee-rye).

Why do you hate him so much?
Anata wa naze kare ga sonna ni dai kirai desu ka?
(An-nah-tah wah nah-zay kah-ray ga soan-nah nee die
kee-rye dess kah?)

Heart—*Kokoro* (Koe-koe-roe).
In matters of love, the heart is often expressed as *mune* (muu-
nay) or "chest."

My heart really thumps when you kiss me.
Anata no kisu de mune ga doki-doki shimasu.
(Ah-nah-tah no kee-sue day muu-nay gah doe-kee-doe-kee
she-mahss).

He turns me on—*Kare wa ikasu wa yo!* (Kah-ray wah ee-kah-sue wah yoe!).

> Does he really get to you that much?
> *Kare wa sonna ni ki ni saseru?*
> (Kah-ray wah soan-nah nee kee nee sah-say-rue?)

Henpecked husband—*Kakadenka no teishu* (Kah-kah dane-kah no tay-e-shoe).
The following colloquial phrase means the same thing and is much more expressive: *Nyobo no shiri ni shikareta otto* (N'yoe-boe no she-ree ni she-kah-ray-tah oat-toe) or "a husband who is under his wife's buttocks."

Hickey—*Kisu maku* (Kee-sue mah-kuu).
This, of course, is from the English "kiss mark." It used to be common for Japanese girls to kiss their lovers as a means of "branding" them, and young men would mark their conquests as a sign of their own virility as well as in the masculine belief that they were providing their girls with a "badge of honor." Hoodlums recruiting young girls for prostitution would also kiss mark them as a visible sign that they had had sex relations. The kiss mark had its heyday in the 1960s, but is still seen (often covered by a neat, white neck bandage), and many young women take pride in being seen with their necks marked.

Highball—*Haiboru* (Hie-boe-rue).
To drink at a hostess bar without hostesses in attendance: *iroke nuki de nomu* (Ee-roe-kay nuu-kee day no-muu). Drink that gives sexual energy: *mamushi faito* (mah-muu-she fie-toe). This latter drink is o'sake in which a mamushi snake has been pickled. **To drink and womanize** – *O'sakeya onna ni kotte iru* (Oh-sah-kay-yah own-nah nee kote-tay ee-rue).

Hips—*Koshi* (Koe-she).
To wiggle the hips, as in sexual intercourse: *Koshi wo igokasu* (Koe-she oh oo-go-kah-sue).

Well! Move your butt!
Sa! Koshi wo ugokase!
(Sah! Koe-she oh ee-go-kah-say!)

Homosexual—*Homo* (Hoe-moe).
Also, *okama* (oh-kah-mah), and *fagu* (fah-guu).

Honeymoon—*Shinkon ryoko* (Sheen-koan rio-koe).

Where are you going on your honeymoon?
Shinkon ryoko wa doko e iku no desu ka?
(Sheen-koan rio-koe wah doe-koe eh ee-kuu no dess kah?)

Horny—*Sukebe* (Sue-kay-bay).
Foreign men in Japan are stereotyped as *sukebe*.

You're really horny tonight, aren't you!
Komban honto ni sukebe desu, ne!
(Koam-bahn hoan-toe nee sue-kay-bay dess, nay!)

Horny old man—*Sukebe jiji* (Sue-kay-bay jee-jee).
Older men in Japan often maintain their reputations as rakes
well into their 60s and 70s.

I want to become a horny old man.
Sukebe jiji ni naritai desu.
(Sue-kay-bay jee-jee nee nah-ree-tie dess.)

Hostess in a bar—*Hosutesu* (Hos-tay-sue).
Bar madame—*Mama-san* (Mah-mah-sahn). In larger cabarets
or hostess clubs, the hostesses are divided into teams, with
leaders, and will often go by team or club names instead of
their own names. New girls entering the profession are taught
ways to attract and keep steady customers. Hostess fees,
hosutesu ryo (hos-tay-sue rio), are charged by the hour.

How much is the hostess fee?
Hosutesu ryo wa ikura desu ka?
(Hos-tay-sue rio wah ee-kuu-rah dess kah?)

Hot sexually—*Moeru* (Moe-rue).

He is always "hot."
Kare wa itsumo moete imasu.
(Kah-ray wah eet-sue-moe moat-tay ee-mahss.)

Hot spring spa—*Onsen* (Own-sin).
Japan literally bubbles with hot springs, hundreds of which
have been developed into resorts for generations. Over 1,000
have medicinal value. All cater to honeymooners and lovers.

Let's go to a Hakone hot spring next week.
Raishu Hakone no onsen ni ikimasho.
(Rye-shuu Hah-koe-nay no own-sin nee ee-kee-mah-show.)

Hug—*Daku* (Dah-kuu).

Please hug me!
Daite kudasai!
(Die-tay kuu-dah-sie.)

Hug me tighter!
Motto kitsuku daite!
(Moat-toe keet-sue-kuu die-tay!)

Husband—*Shujin* (Shuu-jeen).
The generic term for husbands is *otto* (oat-toe). The word *danna* (dahn-nah), an old term that means something like "master of the house," is also sometimes used lightheartedly in reference to someone else's husband. Another word, *teishu* (tay-e-shuu) is rather low-class and is often used in rural and folk humor.

Husband who is no good in bed—*Dame na teishu* (Dah-may nah tay-e-shuu).
Short-tempered husband—*Ki no mijikai teishu* (Kee no me-jee-kie tay-e-shuu). **Husbands who do not stay out late drinking and carousing**—*Majime na teishu* (Mah-jee-may nah tay-e-shuu). Women in the night-time entertainment trades claim to want a *majime* husband, but when the husbands of other women won't play games with them, they are accused of being unmanly or henpecked.

Where is your husband?
Go-shujin wa doko desu ka?
(Go-shuu-jeen wah doe-koe dess kah?)

My husband is not at home.
Uchi-no hito wa inai desu.
(Uu-chee-no ssh-toe wah ee-nie dess.)

When talking about one's own husband, the term *hito* (person) is often used instead of *shujin* (shuu-jeen); as in *uchi no hito* (uu-chee no ssh-toe), or "my husband."

I

I—*Watakushi* (Wah-tock-she).
This is the "standard" word for "I" and is used by both men and women. But there are other commonly used forms of the same word as well as different words altogether, some masculine and some feminine. *Watakushi* is frequently shortened to *watashi* (wah-tah-she) by both men and women, and to *washi* (wah-she) by men.

Strictly masculine words for "I" are *boku* (boe-kuu) and the common *ore* (oh-ray)—although women, particularly entertainers, sometimes use *boku* for special effect. *Boku* is most commonly used by younger men, but it is common to hear older men use it in informal situations. Mothers often address young sons as "*boku*" at which time it is being used as something like "son." *Ore*, a favorite of boys and men, is used only in very casual and gross situations, particularly when they want to indicate their maleness.

Impotent—*Funo* (Fuu-no).
Also, *impo* (eem-poe). Impotence is said to be less common in Japan than in Western countries, apparently because Japanese men have fewer sexual hangups.

Impudent—*Shitsurei na* (Sheet-sue-ray-e nah).
This word is often heard in clubs and cabarets, where getting fresh with the girls is part of the game.

Inn—*Ryokan* (Rio-khan).
There are over 75,000 inns in Japan, pointing up the fact that the Japanese are still great travelers. Traditionally the *ryokan* based their rates on a per-room basis. Several guests could stay in the same room for the price of the room. This system is now followed only by some inns.

Let's stay at an inn tonight.
Komban ryokan ni tomarimasho.
(Koam-bahn rio-khan nee toe-mah-ree-mah-show.)

Until the advent of Western style hotels in Japan (the first ones in the late 1800s), there were over 125,000 inns in Japan—far more overnight accommodations than in any other country at that time.

J

Jealous—*Yakimochi* (Yah-kee-moe-chee).
Jealous husband—*Yakimochi shujin* (Yah-kee-moe-chee shuu-jeen). Like most sexists, Japanese husbands expect their wives and girlfriends to be faithful to them. **Jealous wife**—*Yakimochi nyobo* (Yah-kee-moe-chee n'yoe-boe). Because Japanese wives were traditionally conditioned to suppress any jealous feelings, those who "broke the rules" frequently appear in historical literature as either heroines or villains. Japanese women married to foreign men are said to be more jealous of their husbands than ordinarily.

He is a very jealous husband.
Kare wa yakimochi yaki no otto desu.
(Kah-ray wah yah-kee-moe-chee yah-kee noh oat-toe dess.)

K

Kawasaki—*Kawasaki* (Kah-wah-sah-kee).
This is a city between Tokyo and Yokohama that is noted for its factories and for what are often rated as the best soaplands (massage parlors) in Japan, including several that cater specifically to foreign customers. The soaplands are concentrated in the Horinouchi (Hoe-ree-no-uu-chee) section of Kawasaki.

Kiss—*Kisu* (Kee-sue).

To kiss – *Kisu suru* (Kee-sue sue-rue). The Japanese word for kiss is *seppun* (sape-pune), but is hardly used anymore.

May I kiss you?
Kisu shitemo ii desu ka?
(Kee-sue ssh-tay-moh ee dess kah?)

Kiss me, quick!
Hayaku, kisu shite!
(Hah-yah-kuu kee-sue ssh-tay!)

Kiss me once more before you go.
Wakareru mae ni mo ichido kisu shite.
(Wah-kah-ray-rue my nee moh ee-chee doh kee-sue
ssh-tay.)

Knock up, impregnate—*Ninshin saseru* (Neen-sheen sah-say-rue).

Also, *haramaseru* (hah-rah-mah-say-rue).

He got that girl pregnant.
Kare wa sono onna-no-ko wo haramaseta.
(Kah-ray wah soe-no own-nah-no-koe oh
hah-rah-mah-say-tah)

Kyoto beauty—*Kyoto bijin* (K'yoe-toe bee-jeen).

Kyoto is another area of Japan that has long been famous for beautiful women.

You are really a 'Kyoto beauty,' aren't you!
Anata wa honto ni Kyoto bijin desu ne!
(Ah-nah-tah wah hoan-toe nee K'yoe-toe bee-jeen dess, nay!)

Kyoto bijin is often shortened to *Kyo bijin*.

L

Lady—*FuJin* (Fuu-jeen).
This word is primarily used in formal situations among or about upper-class people. **Lady Tanaka** – *Tanaka Fujin* (Tah-nah-kah fuu-jeen).

Lecherous—*Sukebe* (Sue-kay-bay).
Lechery seems to have been as much admired as condemned during Japan's long feudal period.

Why are girls fascinated by lecherous men?
Onna-no-hito wa naze sukebe na otoko ga suki nano desu ka?
(Own-nah-no-ssh-toe wah nah-zay sue-kay-bay nah
oh-toe-koe ga ski nah-no dess kah?)

Lesbian—*Rezubien* (Ray-zuu-bee-in).
Also, *rezu* (ray-zuu).

Nightclub strippers in Japan are often lesbians.
Naito kurabu no sutorippa ni wa rezu ga oii desu
(Nie-toe kuu-rah-buu no sue-toe-reep-pah nee wah ray-zuu
gah oh-ee-e dess)

Lewd, obscene—*Eichi* (A-e-chee).
This made-up word is taken from the first letter of *hentai sei* (hane-tie say) or "abnormal sex"—in other words, "H" pronounced in Japanese.

Be careful! He is sexually abnormal.
Chui shite! Anohito wa eichi desu.
(Chuu-ee ssh-tay! Ah-nossh-toe wah a-e-chee dess.)

Libertine—*Shikima* (She-kee-mah).

He is a genuine libertine.
Kare wah honto no shikima desu.
(Kah-ray wah hoan-toe no she-kee-mah dess.)

Lie, untruth—*Uso* (Uu-soe). **A liar**—*Usotsuki* (Uu-soat-ski).

You are a liar!
Anata wa usotsuki da yo!
(Ah-nah-tah wah uu-soat-ski dah yoe!)

Like, be fond of—*Suki* (Ski).

I like this.
Kore ga suki desu.
(Koe-ray gah ski dess.)

Do you like Japanese girls?
Anata wa Nihonjin no onna-no-ko ga suki desu ka?
(Ah-nah-tah wah Nee-hoan-jeen no own-nah-no-koe ga ski dess kah?)

Little finger—*Ko yubi* (Koe yuu-bee).
In Japanese sign language, the little finger held up indicates women, or girlfriend, depending on the context. If someone says they are going out and holds up a little finger, it means they are going to meet a girl friend, boyfriend or lover.

Live together out of wedlock—*Dosei suru* (Doe-say sue-rue).

They are living together (even though they are not married).
Anohito-tachi wa dosei shite imasu.
(Ah-no-ssh-toe-tah-chee wah doe-say ssh-tay ee-mahss).

This is a polite way of saying "shack up."

Love—*Ai* (Aye).
To love—*Ai suru* (Aye sue-rue). **To be in love**—*Koi suru* (Koy sue-rue). **Affectionate love**—*Aijo* (Aye-joe). **Love-sick**—*Koi-wazurai* (Koy-wah-zuu-rye).

I love you.
Boku wa anata wo aishite imasu.
(Boe-kuu wah ah-nah-tah oh aye-ssh-tay ee-mahss).

Do you love me?
Anata wa boku wo aishite imasu ka?
(Ah-nah-tah wah boe-kuu oh aye-ssh-tay ee-mahss kah?)

Love affair—*Renai kankei* (Rane-aye kahn-kay-e).
Also, *joji* (joe-jee); *iro-goto* (ee-roe-go-toe). **Love-child**—
Shisei-ji (She-say-e-jee). **Love letter**—*Rabu reta* (Rah-buu
ray-tah). Also *koi bumi* (koy buu-me). **Fake love**—*iroji-kake*
(Ee-roe-jee kah-kay).

Love hotel—*Rabu hoteru* (Rah-buu hoe-tay-rue).
Also, *tsurekomi hoteru* (t'sue-ray-koe-me hoe-tay-rue). **Love
inn**—*Tsurekomi ya* (T'sue-ray-koe-me yah). There are
thousands of inns and hotels in Japan that cater to trysting
couples, usually by the hour.

Lovely—*Airashii* (Aye-rah-she-e).

She is a lovely woman.
Kanojo wa airashii onna desu.
(Kah-no-joe wah aye-rah-she-e own-nah dess.)

Love marriage—*Renai kekkon* (Rane-aye keck-kone).
Over 70 percent of the marriages in Japan today are *renai
kekkon*.

Love potion—*Hore gusuri* (Hoe-ray guu-sue-ree).

Why don't you try a love potion?
Doshite hore gusuri wo shiyo shimasen ka?
(Doh-ssh-tay hoe-ray guu-sue-ree oh she-yoe she-mah-sin
kah?)

Love umbrella—*Aiai gasa* (Aye-aye gah-sah).
Literally "love-love umbrella," this is a large umbrella built
for two—traditionally of beautifully colored oil-paper and
bamboo. You can get some mileage out of having an unusually
large umbrella and offering to share it with a girl when it
suddenly starts to rain.

Love story—*Ai no monogatari* (Aye no moe-no-gah-tah-ree).
Also, *iro banashi* (ee-roe bah-nah-she-e), which has a stronger
sexual connotation. **Love of an older man for a young
woman**—*Oiraku no koi* (Oh-ee-rah-kuu no koy).

Most young Japanese girls love love stories.
*Nihonjin no wakai onna-no-ko wa taitei ai no monogatari
wo konomimasu.*
(Ne-hoan-jeen no wah-kie own-nah-no-koe wah tie-tay-e
aye no moe-no-gah-tah-ree oh koe-no-me-mahss).

Lust—*Shikiyoku* (She-kee-yoe-kuu).
Lustful – *Koshoku* (Koe-show-kuu).

M

Maid—*Meido* (May-e-doe).
Also, *O-ne-san* (Oh-nay-sahn), which actually means "older
sister"; and, *jochu* (joe-chuu), the traditional Japanese word.
O-ne-san is most often used in inns, bars, and restaurants,
when it is synonymous with "waitress." In hotels, *meido* is
commonly used.

Make a pass at—*Iiyoru* (Ee-yoe-rue).
Also, *kudoku* (kuu-doe-kuu).

Make love—*Meku rabu* (May-kuu rah-buu).
Like so many other English words, these have been Japanized
and are generally understood.

> Let's make love.
> *Meku rabu shimasho.*
> (May-kuu rah-buu she-mah-show).

Male—*Dansei* (Dahn-say-e).
This is male in the masculine gender, as in "male sex." It is
also used in tbe sense of men or young men, in reference to
fashions, toilets, etc.

Man—*Otoko* (Oh-toe-koe).
Also, *otoko-no-hito* (oh-toe-koe-no-ssh-toe), which makes it
more specific (as opposed to generic). **Manly**—*Otoko-rashii*
(Oh-toe-koe-rah-she-e). **Unmanly**—*Otoko-rashikunai* (Oh-
toe-koe-rah-she-kuu-nie). **Man talk**—*Otoko-no hanashi* (Oh-
toe-koe-no hah-nah-she). **Man's sexual peak**—*Otoko zakari*
(Oh-toe-koe zah-kah-ree). Unfortunately, men's sexual peak
is during the years when they are still considered boys, 16 to
20. **Man who is strong at night**—*Yoru ni tsuyoi otoko* (Yoe-
rue nee t'sue-yoe-e oh-toe-koe)

Marriage—*Kekkon* (Keck-kone).
Marriage ceremony—*Kekkon shiki* (keck-kone she-kee).
Marriage ceremonies in Japan are usually held in special

marriage halls, in hotel banquet rooms, or large restaurants. It is common for friends and family to tease couples who have been married for only a few months by referring to their marriage as still "sexually hot" or still in the honeymoon stage: *shinkon hoya hoya* (sheen-kone hoe-yah hoe-yah). Mixed-marriages (Japanese-foreign) are called *zakkon* (zack-kone).

Marry—*Kekkon suru* (Keck-kone sue-rue).

Are you married?
Anata wa kekkon shite imasu ka?
(Ah-nah-tah wah keck-kone ssh-tay ee-mahss-kah?)

I'm not married.
Kekkon shite nai.
(Keck-kone ssh-tay nie).

She wants to marry for money.
Kanojo wa okane meate no kekkon ga shitai desu
(Kah-no-joe wah oh-kah-nay may-ah-tay no keck-kone ga she-tie dess.)

Massage—*Masaji* (Mah-sah-jee).

In Japan massage is usually associated with sex.
Nihon de wa masaji to sekusu ga taitei kankei shite imasu.
(Nee-hoan day wah mah-sah-jee toe say-kuu-sue gah tie-tay-e kahn-kay-e ssh-tay ee-mahss).

Masturbation by male—*Senzuri suru* (Sen-zuu-ree sue-rue).
Masturbation by female—*manzuri suru* (mahn-zuu-ree sue-rue). **Masturbate to excess**—*Kokisugi suru* (Koe-kee-sue-ghee sue-rue). Also, **masturbation**—*masutabeshon* (mahss-tah-bay-shoan); also, *masu wo kaku* (mah-sue oh kah-kuu); and *onani* (oh-nah-nee). Soaplands now offer masturbation as one of their tension-relieving services.

Mature about sexual matters—*Maseteiru* (Mah-say-tay-ee-rue).

Even though she is young, she knows a lot about sex.
Kanojo wa wakai kedo masete imasu.
(Kah-no-joe wah wah-kie kay-doe mah-say-tay ee-mahss.)

Meeting place—*Au basho* (Ow bah-show).

Do you know a good meeting place on the Ginza?
Ginza de ii au basho wo shitte imasu ka?
(Geen-zah day ee ow bah-show oh ssh-tay ee-mahss kah?)

Mistress—*Omekake* (Oh-may-kah-kay).
This literally means "one on whom you hang your eyes," apparently in reference to the fact that most mistresses are good to look at. Also, *ni-go-san* (nee-go-sahn) or "Mrs. Number Two." Mistress-keeping is still a common custom in Japan.

"Morning sex"—*Asappara kara no sekusu* (Ah-sap-pah-rah kah-rah no say-kuu-sue).
Also, *moningu sekusu* (moe-neen-guu say-kuu-sue).

Some people say morning sex is the best.
Aru hito wa moningu sekusu ga ichiban ii to iimasu.
(Ah-rue ssh-toe wah moe-neen-guu say-kuu-sue gah ee-
chee-bahn ee to ee-mahss).

Motel—*Moteru* (Moe-tay-rue).
With the development of recreational driving in Japan in the
1960s and 70s, roadside motels proliferated. They now
compete with traditional inns and urban lov-tels as popular
trysting places. Most motels offer rooms on a two-hour basis
for this purpose. Veteran users select different motels
according to their decor and "mood."

N

Nag—*Kuchi yakamashii* (Kuu-chee yah-kah-mah-she-e).

My friend's wife is always nagging him.
*Boku no tomodachi no oku-san ga itsumo kuchi
yakamashii desu.*
(Boe-kuu no toe-moe-dah-chee no oak-san gah eet-sue-moe
kuu-chee yah-kah-mah-she-e dess.)

Naked—*Hadaka* (Hah-dah-kah).
Stark naked—*Mappadaka* (Mop-pah-dah-kah). A famous
Canadian male singer was once caught *mappadaka* chasing
a Japanese girl down the hallway of one of Tokyo's luxury
hotels. He was not arrested, apparently because he was
"properly dressed" for the sport he was engaged in.

Nasty—*Iyarashii* (Eyah-rah-she-e).
When men use sexual or vulgar language to women, particularly in the hostess world, the girls often tell the men they are *iyarashii*—in a manner that is usually more complimentary than critical.

Need—*Hitsuyo* (Heet-sue-yoh).

I need you!
Anata ga hitsuyo desu!
(Ah-nah-tah gah heet-sue-yoh dess!)

Nice—*Suteki* (Sue-tay-kee).

Isn't that a nice dress!
Ma! Suteki na doresu desu, ne!
(Mah! Sue-tay-kee nah doe-ray-sue dess, nay!)

You (it) look(s) (is) nice!
Suteki desu yo!
(Sue-tay-kee dess yo!)

Night cap—*Ne-zake* (Nay-zah-kay).
Ne (Nay) is sleep and *zake* (zah-kay) is alcoholic drink.
Morning drink—*Asa zake* (Ah-sah zah-kay).

Nightclub—*Naito kurahu* (Nie-toe kuu-rah-buu).
The difference between a nightclub and cabaret in Japan is that in nightclubs patrons have a choice of whether or not to have hostesses join them, and nightclubs usually have live

entertainment while cabarets, unless they are quite large, generally do not. Couples are also welcome at nightclubs. In cabarets it is customarily men only.

Nightcrawling—*Yohai* (Yoe-hi).

Prior to the 19th century in rural Japan a popular courting system was for young men to surreptitiously enter the homes of the girls of their choice at night and crawl into bed with them. The practice in the countryside has disappeared but the word is still known and used in a humorous manner. There are, however, instances of *yohai* during company outings when male and female employees by the dozens put up at resort inns for two or three nights of revelry.

Night girl—*Yoru no onna* (Yoe-rue no own-nah).

A *yoru no onna* is one who works at night, usually in the entertainment trades, and possibly as a prostitute. Another old term is *yoru no cho* (yoe-rue no choe) or "night-time butterfly"—in other words, a woman who flits from man to man at night.

Night play—*Yo asobi* (Yoe ah-so-bee).

Drinking and philandering in Japan's huge and thriving world of bars, clubs, and cabarets is known appropriately as *yo asobi* or "night play." The connotation is definitely sexual.

Nipple—*Chikubi* (Chee-kuu-bee).

No!—*Irya da!* (E-yah dah!).
This is what a woman says to a man when he is trying to force his attentions on her. It is also used when a woman is being very emphatic in turning down a proposition.

Nude—*Nudo* (Nuu-doe).
Also, *hadaka-no* (hah-dah-kah-no). **Nude heaven**—*Hadaka tengoku* (Hah-dah-kah tane-go-kuu). Hot spring spa baths in resort areas, where the sexes generally bathe together, are sometimes referred to as *hadaka tengoku*.

Nude studio—*Nudo sutajio* (Nuu-doe stah-jee-oh).
Nude studios, where men pay a fee to photograph (or pretend to photograph) naked women, date from the closing of the red-light districts in 1956–57. The only ones remaining are usually found in the sleazier bar districts.

Nymphomania—*Joshi-iransho* (Joe-she-ee-rahn-show).
Also, *shiki-joku* (she-kee-joe-kuu).

O

Obi—*Obi* (Oh-bee).
This is the wide sash wrapped around the kimono and *yukata* to keep them closed. One of Japan's most popular folk songs refers to whether or not a young man is manly enough to get a girl to undo her *obi*.

One-shot—*Ippatsu* (Eep-pot-sue).
Usually refers to one sexual encounter or climax. Also, *ippatsu no otoko* (eep-pot-sue no oh-toe-koe), or a man who can climax only once over a long period of time.

One man in bed with two women—*Uguisu-no taniwatari* (Uu-guu-ee-suu-no tah-nee-wah-tah-ree).
Literally: a nightingale flying back and forth over a narrow valley. An old term, but one that most people still understand.

One-way love—*Kata-omoi* (Kah-tah-oh-moe-e).
This is "one-way thinking," in reference to someone loving a person who doesn't return the feeling.

Orgy—*Ranko paati* (Rahn-koe pah-tee).

Let's have a sex orgy!
Ranko paati shimasho!
(Rahn-koe pah-tee she-mah-show!)

Over-do-it—*Yari sugimasu* (Yah-ree suu-ghee-mahss).
I over did it (sex, etc.)—*Yari sugimashita* (Yah-ree-sue-ghee-mahssh-tah). **I over-drank**—*Nomi sugimashita* (No-me sue-ghee-mahssh-tah). **I over-ate**—*Tabe sugimashita* (Tah-bay sue-ghee-mahssh-tah).

P

Panties—*Panti* (Pahn-tee).
Panty thief—*Pahn-tee dorobo* (pahn-tee doe-roe-boe). In Japan some men get hung up on stealing the panties of young girls and women. Pull down one's **panties**—*Panti wo sageru* (Pahn-tee oh sah-gay-rue).

> Take your panties off.
> *Panti wo nuide.*
> (Pahn-tee oh nuu-e-day).

Paramour—*Jofu* (Joe-fuu).

> She is the paramour of a wealthy businessman.
> *Kanojo wa kanemochi gyosha no jofu desu.*
> (Kah-no-joe wab kah-nay-moe-chee g'yoe-shah no
> joe-fuu dess.)

Passion—*Jonetsu* (Joe-nate-sue).
Passionate—*Jonetsu-teki* (Joe-nate-sue-tay-kee). **Passionate look**—*Iro me* (Ee-roe may). "**Passion lobes**"—*Mimi tabu ga okii* (Me-me tah-buu gah oh-kee-e). In Japan (and China) long, large earlobes are regarded as a sign of strong sexuality and stamina.

"**Passion lip**"—*Hana no shita ga nagai* (Hah-nah no ssh-tah gah nah-guy).
When the space between the upper lip and the nose is large and the upper lip is well-grooved, it is regarded as another

sign of unusual sexuality. Men who are sexually aggressive are often accused of having a *hana no shita ga nagai* even when it isn't especially long.

When one is obviously or believed to be thinking about sex, he or she may be described as *hana no shita wo nobasu* (Hah-nah no ssh-tah oh no-bah-sue) or "lengthening the space beneath the nose."

She is a passionate woman.
Kanojo wa taihen jonetsu-teki na onna desu.
(Kah-no-joe wab tie-hane joe-nate-sue-tay-kee nah
own-nah dess.)

I was overcome with passion.
Boku wa chiho ni oboremashita.
(Boe-kuu wab chee-hoe nee oh-boe-ray-mahssh-tah).

Penis—*Inkei* (Inn-kay-e).

This is the medical term for the male whang. Among the dozen or so colloquial and slang words for the same thing: *chimpo* (cheem-poe); *O-chin-chin* (Oh-cheen-cheen); *dankon* (dahn-kohn), which means "male root"; *dansei jishin* (dabn-say-e jee-sheen), or "male confidence"; *meru shimboru* (may-rue sheem-boe-rue), "male symbol"; *pinesu* (pee-nay-sue); *ichi butsu* (ee-chee boot-sue), "the one thing"; *are* (ah-ray) or "that"; *mara* (mah-rah), which might be translated as "round thing," etc.

Among these, *chimpo* or *chimbo* is probably the most commonly used. Men who have had intercourse with the same woman used to be known as *mara kyodai* (mah-rah k'yoe-die) or "brothers of the prick."

Perfume—*Kosui* (Koe-sue-e).

Your perfume really turns me on.
Anata no kosui wa boku wo kofun sasemasu.
(Ah-nah-tab no koe-sue-e wah boe-kuu oh koe-fuun
sah-say-mahss).

Japanese women, as a rule, do not like to wear a lot of perfume, preferring the power of subtlety.

Pervert, sexual—*Chikan* (Chee-kahn).
Men who fondle women on crowded trains and subways are called *chikan*.

Philanderer—*Uwakimono* (Uu-wab-kee-moe-no).
This is the term usually applied to men. When women philander it is usually called *yoromeku* (yoe-roe-may-kuu).

She had an affair with him.
Kanojo wa kare ni yoromekimashita.
(Kah-no-joe wah kah-ray nee yoe-roe-may-kee-mahssh-tah).

Pimples—*Nikibi* (Nee-kee-bee).
Pimple-faced—*Nikibidarake* (Nee-kee-bee-dah-rah-kay).
Before young Japanese boys and girls started eating American-style foods and drinking soft drinks, they seldom (if ever!) had pimples.

Pimp—*Ponbiki* (Pahn-bee-kee).

Pitiful—*Kawaiso* (Kah-wah-e-soe). An often used word in male-female relations, particularly in the "water business" trade, where cabaret hostesses are so ready to commiserate with customers who complain about their wives, their lovelife, or their business.

> That's a shame! You are to be pitied!
> *Kawaiso desu, ne!*
> (Kah-wah-e-soe dess, nay!)

Playgirl—*Pureigaru* (Puu-ray-e-gah-rue). Also, an old Japanese word: *abazure* (ah-bah-zuu-ray).

Pornographic photos—*Ero shashin* (Eh-roe shah-sheen).
Pornographic arts—*Shun ga* (Shune gah), or "spring arts."

Pornography—*Poruno* (Poe-rue-no).
The Japanese distinguish between stylized traditional "Japanese" pornography and foreign porn. Most modern-day Japanese porn is made up of black-and-white line drawings published in comic-book form. Foreign porn magazines are usually censored.

Pregnant—*Ninshin* (Neen-sheen).
To become pregnant—*Ninshin suru* (Neen-sheen sue-rue). Also, *onaka ga okii* (oh-nah-kah gah oh-kee-e). The latter literally means "the stomach is big."

My girlfriend is not pregnant!
Boku no garu furendo wa ninshin shite imasen yo!
(Boe-kuu no gah-rue fuu-ren-doe wah neen-sheen ssh-tay
ee-mah-sen yoe!)

Premarital sex—*Kekkon mae no sekusu* (Keck-kone my no
say-kuu-sue).
Also, the old term, *konzen kosho* (kone-zen koe-show).

Premature ejaculation—*Soro* (Soe-roe).
Men who ejaculate quickly are often called *haya-uchi* (hah-
yah-uu-chee), the Japanese equivalent of "quick on the draw"
or "fast shooter."

Pretty—*Kirei* (Kee-ray-e).
Pretty girl—*Kirei na onnanoko* (Kee-ray-e nah own-nah-no-
koe).

That is really a pretty girl.
Anohito wa honto ni kirei na onnanoko desu
(Ah-no-ssh-toe wah hoan-toe nee kee-ray-e nah own-nah-
no-koe dess.)

Pretty eyes—*Kirei na me* (Kee-ray-ee nah may).

Your eyes are pretty.
Anata no me wa kirei desu
(Ah-nah-tah no may wah kee-ray-ee dess.)

Pretty hair—*Kirei na kami* (Kee-ray-e nah kah-me).
Pretty legs—*Kirei na ashi* (Kee-ray-e nah ah-she).

You are the prettiest girl in the world.
Anata wa sekai-ichi no bijin desu.
(Ah-nah-tah wah say-kie-ee-chee no bee-jeen dess.)

"Private parts"—*Kyoku bu* (K'yoe-kuu buu).
Also, *im bu* (emm buu). If the female attendant in a soapland washes your "private parts" for you, it is a sign that other services are also available.

Promiscuous woman—*Shin no karui onna* (She-ree no kah-rue-e own-nah).
Literally, "a woman whose rear end is lightweight"—that is, moves around easily from man to man. An old term, but using it will make you sound really deep—or weird!

Propose marriage—*Propozu* (Pro-poe-zuu).
The Japanese word, now seldom heard, is *kyukon suru* (Que-kone sue-rue).

I am going to propose to my girlfriend.
Garu furendo ni propozu shimasu.
(Gah-rue fuu-ren-doe nee pro-poe-zuu she-mahss).

Prostitute—*Shofu* (Show-fuu).

Also, *panpan* (pahn-pahn), and *pamma* (pom-mah), from *panpan* and *amma* (ahm-mah), or masseuse, in reference to massage women who double as prostitutes. The formal word for prostitute is *baishunfu* (by-shune-fuu). Foreign prostitutes make out especially well in Japan if they are young, blonde, and busty, in that order.

Prostitution—*Baishun* (By-shune).

This word literally means to "sell spring," spring being a euphemism for sex. Prostitution was legal in Japan until April Fool's Day, 1957. It was outlawed on April 1, 1956, with a one-year grace period for brothel operators and prostitutes to switch to new occupations.

Puberty – *Toshigoro* (Toe-she-go-roe).

To reach puberty – *Iro ke zuku* (Ee-roe kay zuu-kuu).

Pubic hair—*Immo* (Emm-moe).

Also the Japanized English *hea* (hay-ah), and the colloquial term *shigemi* (she-gay-me). Male pubic hair is also called *chin ke* (cheen kay). Some Japanese men and women have great shocks of pubic hair; others very little. Copius pubic hair on a man is regarded as masculine—or animalistic if the man is crudely aggressive. Women with an unusual amount of pubic hair tend to be stereotyped as "man-like" or unrefined and sexually wanton. There is a song (or poem) about women jumping over burning fires to singe off the excess hair. At the same time, however, especially scanty hair in the pubic area is an embarrassment to both men and women (and it is wise not to mention it). Other words referring to female pubic hair: *junguru* (jahn-guu-rue) from jungle; and *deruta* (day-rue-tah) from delta.

Public bath—*Sento* (Sin-toe).
Japan's once common public bathhouses have continued to shrink in numbers as more and more people have private baths or showers in their homes. The baths were segregated by sex in the early 1950s, but in many bathhouses one can peer into the undressing areas of the opposite sex when "checking in."

R

Rape—*Gokan suru* (Go-khan sue-rue).

She was raped by two hoodlums.
Kanojo wa futari no gurentai ni gokan saremashita.
(Kah-no-joe wah fuu-tah-ree no guu-ren-tie nee go-khan sah-ray-mahssh-tah.)

Rear end—*Oshiri* (Oh-she-ree).
Also, *ketsu* (kate-sue), which is a vulgar word comparable to "ass." Rear view of a woman with a seductive behind: *Bakkushan* (Bach-kuu-shawn).

Who pinched my girl's rear end?
Dare ga boku no kanojo no oshiri wo tsunerimashita ka?
(Dah-ray gah boe-kuu no kah-no-joe no oh-she-ree oh t'sue-nay-ree-mahssh-tah kah?)

Generally speaking, comments about the *oshiri* are not regarded as vulgar (insulting, maybe, but not vulgar), as in the usage of "butt."

Red-light district—*Akasen chitai* (Ah-kah-sin chee-tie).
Another word that has long been associated with red-light districts in Japan is *asagaeri* (ah-sah-guy-ree), which means "returning home in the morning" (after a night in a whorehouse). It is still used in a humorous manner in reference to staying out all night at love hotels or love inns, etc.

Right to choose—*Erabu kenri* (Eh-rah-buu ken-ree).
Repeat customers at cabarets and soaplands, etc., have "the right to choose" the girls they want. This term is also used in other, non "water business" occasions as well.

Romance – *Romansu* (Roe-mahn-sue).
Young Japanese, especially girls, are very romantic-minded. Girls react strongly to romantic behavior by men. **"Big romance"**—*Saiko no romansu* (Sie-koe no roe-mahn-sue). **Romance gray**—*Romansu gurei* (Roe-mahn-sue guu-ray-e)—referring to an older man with gray hair having a romance with a young woman.

Old Japanese words with similar meanings: *koi-ji* (koy-jee); *rei-ai* (ray-e-aye); *iro-goto* (ee-roe-go-toe). The latter word is more sexually tinged than the others.

His mind is always on romance.
Kare wa itsumo iro-goto bakari wo kangaete imasu.
(Kah-ray wah eet-sue-moe ee-roe-go-toe bah-kah-ree oh
kahn-guy-tay ee-mahss.)

Room—*Heya* (Hay-yah).
Room rate—*Heya dai* (Hay-yah die). Rooms in lov-tels and love inns are usually rented by the hour. There is usually an extra charge for the use of hot baths in love inns.

Rubber condom—*Kondommu* (Kone-doe-muu).
Also, *gomu* (go-muu), meaning "rubber"; and *saku* (sah-kuu), from the English "sack." In earlier years, *herumetto* (hay-rue-may-toe) or "helmet" was also used.

Shall I use a condom?
Kondommu wo tsukaimasho ka?
(Kone-doe-muu oh t'sue-kie-mah-show kah?)

Don't you have a rubber?
Gomu ga arimasen ka?
(Go-muu gah ah-ree-mah-sin kah?)

S

Sad—*Kanashii* (Kah-nah-she-e).
Sad-faced—*Kanashii kao* (Kah-nah-she-e kah-oh).

Why are you sad?
Naze kanashii no desu ka?
(Nah-zay kah-nah-she-e no dess kah?)

Sad story—*Itamashii monogatari* (Ee-tah-mah-shee moe-no-gah-tah-ree).
Women who work in the entertainment trades often tell their customers sad stories to make them more generous and less sexually aggressive. Many of the stories are true but patrons who are taken in by them often lose more than their pants.

Saké—*Saké* (sah-kay).
Often with an honorific "O" as a prefix: O'saké. This is the traditional wine-like Japanese drink made from rice. It is also often used in a generic sense referring to all alcoholic drinks. To specify saké, say *Nihon-shu* (Nee-hoan shuu). **Sake cup** —*saka zuki* (sah-kah zuu-kee). **Saké decanter** (for heating it)—*tokkuri* (toke-kuu-ree). **Top-grade sake**—*Tokkyu shu* (Toke-que shuu); **First-grade saké**—*Eek-kyu shu* (Ee-que shuu). **Second-grade saké**—*Nikyu shu* (Nee-que shuu).

"Science of Pubic Hair"—*Mogaku* (Moe-gah-kuu).
In the 1950s a Japanese professor made an exhaustive study of the relationship between the shape and quality of female

pubic hair and the personality and sexual inclinations of the women. He called his new field of study *mogaku* or "science of pubic hair," raising more than a few eyebrows when he published his work. Check it out. (A clear triangle shape is preferred.)

Secret (love) rendezvous—*Aibiki* (Aye-bee-kee).
An *aibiki* is usually with a lover one is seeing secretly. It is an old word, used in Japan before 1945 when open dating was not socially sanctioned. Using it today can get some interesting results.

Sensual—*Kannoteki* (Kahn-no-tay-kee).
Sensuous—*Nikukanteki* (Nee-kuu-kahn-tay-kee).

She is a very sensual woman.
Kanojo wa kannoteki na onna desu.
(Kah-no-joe wah kahn-no-tay-kee nah own-nah dess.)

Seven-year-itch—*Shichi-nen-me no kayumi* (She-chee-nane-may no kah-yuu-me).
This is a direct translation from the English. A Japanized version: *shichi-nen-me no uwaki* (she-chee-nane-may no uu-wah-kee).

Sex—*Sei* (Say-e). Also, *sekusu* (say-kuu-sue).
The sex act—*Seiko* (Say-e koe). **Sex appeal**—*Sei teki* (Say-e tay-kee). **Sex crazy**—*Iro kichigai* (Ee-roe kee-chee-guy). **Sex life**—*Sei seikatsu* (Say-e say-e-kot-sue). **Sex movie**—Ero dakushon (A-roe dah-kuu-shone). **Sex party**—*Sekusu paati*

(Say-kuu-sue pah-tee). **Sex pervert**—*Hentai seiyokusha* (Hane-tie say-e-yoke-shah). **Sex problem**—*Sei mondai* (Say-e moan-die). **Sex education**—*Sei kyoiku* (Say-e k'yoe-ee-kuu).

How's your sex life?
Anata no sei seikatsu wa doh desu ka?
(Ah-nah-tah no say-e say-e-kot-sue wah doh dess kah?)

Sexual—*Seiteki* (Say-e-tay-kee).
Sexual appetite—*Sei yoku* (Say-e yoe-kuu). Also, *sei-ryoku* (say-e rio-kuu). **Sexual energy**—*Sekusu no sutamina* (Say-kuu-sue no stah-me-nah). **Have sexual intercourse**—*Seiko wo suru* (Say-e-koe oh sue-rue). **Sexual addiction**—*Iro ni tandeki suru* (Ee-roe nee tahn-day-kee sue-rue).

He is addicted to sex.
Kare wa iro ni tandeki shite imasu.
(Kah-ray wah ee-roe nee tahn-day-kee ssh-tay ee-mahss.)

Sexual morality—*Sei dotoku* (Say-e doe-toe-kuu).
Sexual passion—*Shikijo* (She-kee joe). **"Sexual service"**—*Sekushuaru sabisu* (Say-kuu-shu-ahl sah-bee-sue). When referring to a cabaret setting, "sexual service" refers to hostesses letting patrons touch and fondle them—not to sexual intercourse or other forms of sexual activity.

There is a strong element of "infantile sexuality" in Japanese sexual behavior, both male and female. It embodies a kind of behavior marked by passive dependence and a baby-like helplessness that is an essential part of interpersonal relations in Japan. This type of behavior is frequently used by women to turn men on, and by men to get women to "mother" or "baby" them. Girls and women using this approach may also talk in "baby" voices, act childish, and appear sexually vulnerable.

Sexy man—*Irogoto shi* (Ee-roe-go-toe she).
Sexy woman—*Iroppoi onna* (Ee-rope-poy own-nah). An *iroppoi onna* may also mean a prostitute or a mistress in the general sense. **Beautiful woman who is very sensual**—*Nikutai bijin* (Nee-kuu-tie bee-jeen). **Woman who is over-sexed**—*Ijo seiyoku onna* (Ee-joe say-e-yoe-kuu own-nah).

> I would like to meet an over-sexed woman.
> *Boku wa ijo seiyoku onna to aitai desu.*
> (Boe-kuu wa ee-joe say-e-yoe-kuu own-nah toe
> aye-tie dess).

Shack up—*Dosei suru* (Doh-say-e suu-rue).

> I hear she is shacked up with a professor.
> *Kanojo ga kyoju to dosei shite iru so desu.*
> (Kah-no-joe ga k'yoe-juu to doh-say-e ssh-tay ee-rue
> so dess.)

Sixty-nine—*Sikusuti nainu* (See-kuu-stee nie-nuu).
Or in Japanese, *rokuju kyu* (roe-kuu-juu que). In this context, 69 means the same as in English—a man and a woman assume a head-to-genital position to engage in oral sex simultaneously.

Skinny dip – *Furu chin* (Fuu-ruu cheen)
Usually refers to men. Also, *maru dashi* (mah-rue dah-she), which means "displaying the front" and is usually used in reference to women.

Sleeping gown—*Nemaki* (Nay-mah-kee).
This is a lightweight, kimono-styled printed cotton robe used as a sleeping gown and casual around-the-house wear. The *yukata* version of the same thing is used as costume-of-the-day in resort spas and often at neighborhood festivals on holidays and evenings.

Sleep with—*Issho ni neru* (E-show nee nay-rue).

I want to sleep with you.
Watakushi wa anata to netai desu.
(Wah-tock-she wah ah-nah-tah toe nay-tie dess.)

Small—*Chiisai* (Chee-e-sie).
The philosophy of "small is beautiful" has long been a primary factor in Japanese culture. But it doesn't apply to all sexual matters!

Snapping pussy—*Hamaguri* (Hah-mah-guu-ree).
A real *hamaguri* is an edible mussel that snaps shut when something is stuck into it. In this case, it refers to a woman who has learned how to exercise control over the muscles surrounding her vagina, and can grip or massage her lover's *chimpo* after penetration. Another term used in the same way:

kinchaku (keen chah-kuu) which originally referred to a purse with drawstrings.

Soap—*Sekken* (Sake-ken).
Cleanliness is traditional in Japan and is also closely associated with sex—a bath before and after being highly prized.

Soapland—*Soapland.*
These are Japan's hot bath massage parlors (formerly known as Turkish baths), which cater primarily to men looking for sex. There are hundreds of them throughout Japan, with over 200 in Tokyo alone at the last count. Most are located in or near recognized entertainment districts or near major transportation terminals. Some vocabulary used in the baths: *homban* (home-bahn), meaning "the real thing" or straight sexual intercourse; *ofera* (oh-fay-rah) and *shakuhachi* (shah-kuu-hah-chee), both referring to oral sex; and *Awa Odori* (Ah-wah Oh-doe-ree), a folk dance that originated in the Awa district of Japan, but in this context refers to a bathhouse girl soaping down the customer's body by soaping herself, then slithering all over the customer while both are on an air mattress. *Awa* also means "soap bubbles," so the expression may be translated as "soap bubble dance."

Osupe (Oh-sue-pay), short for "special," refers to the female attendant masturbating the customer. *Daburu osupe* (Dah-buu-rue oh-suu-pay), or "double special," also a 69er—reversing ends, the customer and attendant masturbate each other. *Tawashi* (Tah-wah-she), to rub soap on the erogenic zones.

"Sock it to me!"—*Ii wa! Motto yatte!* (Ee, wah! Moat-toe yaht-tay!).

Often said by women when they want to encourage their male partners to put their all into it.

Son—*Musuko* (Muu-sue-koe).

This means "son" in the usual sense, and is also used as a euphemism for the male sex organ. In the "water business" one is likely to hear such things as:

"Your 'son' is really active today, isn't he!"
Kyo wa anata no musuko ga totemo genki desu, ne!
(K'yoe wah ah-nah-tah no muu-sue-koe gah toe-tay-moe
gane-kee dess, nay!)

Another word for son, *segare* (say-gah-ray) is also used in this sexual connotation.

Stag party—*Otoko dake no enkai* (Oh-toe-koe dah-kay no inn-kie).

I'm going to a stag party tonight.
Komban otoko dake no enkai ni ikimasu.
(Komb-bahn oh-toe-koe dah-kay no inn-kie nee
ee-kee-mahss).

Stingy—*Kechi* (Kay-chee).

Hey, tightwad! You forgot your change!
Oi, kechi! Otsuri wo wasuretan da zo!
(Ohh-ee, kay-chee! Oat-sue-ree oh wah-sue-ray-tahn
dah zoe!)

T

Thick-skinned—*Tsura no kawa ga atsui* (T'sue-rah no kah-wah gah aht-sue-e).
This is sometimes used as the equivalent of "bastard" and is usually by women in reference to callous men.

You're really thick-skinned, aren't you!
Tsura no kawa no atsui hito desu, ne!
(T'sue-rah no kah-wah no aht-sue-e ssh-toe dess, nay!)

Thirty-three—*Sati suri* (Sah-tee suu-ree).
This is the Japanese pronunciation of 33, used in reference to a man who is slow to climax—a take-off on the old sluggish 33 rpm record.

Three-sex—*Suri sekusu* (Suu-ree say-kuu-sue).
When three people (usually but not necessarily one man and two women) engage in sexual activities together you have "three sex." Also, *toripuru purei* (toe-ree-puu-ruu puu-ray), or "triple play," from American baseball.

Thumb—*Oyayubi* (Oh-yah-yuu-bee).

The thumb held up by itself means male or boy friend in Japanese sign language.

Titties—*Chichi* (Chee-chee).

In pre-Western influenced Japan, the nape of the neck was considered more sexually titillating than the female breasts. *Chichi* has about the same connotation as "breasts."

Tohoku beauties—*Tohoku bijin* (Toe-hoe-kuu bee-jeen).

The Tohoku district in northern Honshu, Japan's main island, is noted for its big-eyed, light-skinned beautiful women who are known as *Tohoku bijin* or "Tohoku beauties." The reason for this phenomenon is that they have some Ainu genes in the makeup—Ainu being the indigenous Caucasoid race that originally inhabited the central and northern islands of Japan.

Toilet—*Toireto* (Toy-rate-toe).

Also, *o-toire* (oh-toy-e-ray). In addition to these two Japanese pronunciations of the English word "toilet," there are over half a dozen other words, such as *otearai* (oh-tay-ah-rye) or "hand-washing place"; *habakari* (hah-bah-kah-ree); *gojujo* (go-fuu-joe), and *benjo* (bane-joe)—in descending order of politeness. Women mostly use *gofujo* or *otearai*. Men primarily use *otearai* and *benjo*, the latter in informal and gross situations.

Topless—*Topuresu* (Toe-puu-ray-sue).
Toplessness has been old hat in Japan for thousands of years—among nursing mothers, grandmothers cooling themselves in summertime, pearl divers, and users of public baths. Americans taught them how to make a titillating show of it in the late 1940s and 50s.

Triangle relationship—*Sankaku kankei* (Sahn-kah-kuu kahn-kay-e).
This phrase is sometimes used when two men and one woman or one man and two women are involved in a love triangle.

Turns me on sexually—*Kofun saseru* (Koe-fuun sah-say-rue).

She really turns me on.
Kanojo wa honto ni kofun sasemasu.
(Kah-no-jo wah hoan-toe nee koe-fuun sah-say-mahss).

U

Undress—*Yofuku wo nugu* (Yoe-fuu-kuu oh nuu-guu).

Well! It's time to take off your (our) clothes!
Sa! Yofuku wo nugu jikan desu!
(Sah! Yoe-fuu-kuu oh nuu-guu jee-khan dess!)

V

Vagina—*Chitsu* (Cheet-sue).
This is the medical term. A poetic term is *ai-no izumi* (aye-no ee-zuu-mee) or "fountain of love." An old euphemism is *hanagai* (hah-nah-guy), a beautiful colored shell-shaped something like the vagina. A vulgar "four-letter word" type of term: *o-manko* (oh-mahn-koe).

Venereal disease—*Seibyo* (Say-e-b'yoe).
There is also the diminutive, *bai-chan* (by-chahn). In Japan, unlike in the West, penicillin and other antibiotic drugs can be purchased over-the-counter without a prescription, resulting in many people treating themselves for STDs. Not surprisingly, some over-dose and others under-dose.

Virgin—*Shojo* (Show-joe).
Another word: *bajin* (bah-jeen) from the English. During the heyday of the "Floating World" of old Japan well-to-do men often paid large sums for the opportunity to "deflower" newly obtained prostitutes and apprentice geisha. When young geisha had their first sexual intercourse, a traditional ceremony, called *Mizu-Age Shiki* (Me-zoo-Ah-gay She-kee),was conducted. This term means "Water Giving Ceremony."

Voluptuous—*Nikutai-teki* (Nee-kuu-tie-tay-kee).
Also, *shushoku ni oboreta* (shuu-show-kuu nee oh-boe-ray-tah).

I met a very voluptuous woman last night.
Yube taihen nikutai-teki na onna ni aimashita.
(Yuu-bay tie-hane nee-kuu-tie-tay-kee nah own-nah nee
aye-mahssh-tah.)

W

Ward office—*Ku yakusho* (Kuu yahk-show).
The legal portion of marriages in Japan is registering the union
in the local office of the ward (if a large city), village, or
county seat.

"Water business"—*Mizu shobai* (Mee-zuu show-by).
This is a generic term used in reference to all the entertainment
trades that involve hot baths, drinking, and night-time
recreational activities—bars, cabarets, geisha inns, love hotels,
etc. It apparently came about because sexually oriented
businesses in earlier times were usually combined with bathing
facilities.

Wedding—*Kekkon shiki* (Keck-kone she-kee).
Wedding day—*Kekkon no hi* (Keck-kone no he). **Wedding
ring**—*Kekkon yubiwa* (Keck-kone yuu-bee-wah). **Wedding
anniversary**—*Kekkon kinenbi* (Keck-kone kee-nane-bee).

When is your wedding?
Kekkon shiki wa itsu desu ka?
(Keck-kone she-kee wah eet-sue dess kah?)

Wet dream—*Ii yume* (Ee yuu-may).
This literally means a "good dream."

> I had (saw) a wet dream last night.
> *Yube ii yume wo mimashita.*
> (Yuu-bay ee yuu-may oh me-mahssh-tah).

A more formal word for wet dream is *musei* (muu-say).

> I had a wet dream last night.
> *Yube musei shimashita.*
> (Yuu-bay muu-say she-mahssh-tah.)

Whisky—*Uisuki* (Uu-wee-ski).
Whisky with water—*Mizu wari* (Mee-zuu wah-ree), which usually means Scotch and water. **Whisky with soda**—*Soda wari* (Soe-dah wah-ree).

Whore—*Baishunfu* (By-shune-fuu).
Also, the vulgar *pansuke* (pahn-skay). **Wife**—*Oku-san* (Oak-san). There are several words in Japanese for wife, depending on whose wife and the social level of the language being used. Wife in the generic sense is *nyobo* (n'yoe-boe). When talking to someone else's wife or about anyone else's wife the proper term is *oku-san*—which could be literally translated as "Mrs. Honorable Inside." One's own wife is *nyobo* or *kanai* (kah-nie). A bossy wife is a *kampaku nyobo* (kahm-pah-kuu n'yoe-boe)—a term that refers to the shogun during Japan's long feudal age. A "second wife" (mistress) was traditionally called

Ni-go san (Nee-go sahn) or "Mrs. No.2." Affluent men could take a No.3 or more.

Wig—*Katsura* (Kot-sue-rah).
Most Japanese women who wear kimono at their wedding may also wear a traditionally styled wig.

Wine—*Budoshu* (Buu-doe-shuu).
This is wine from grapes (*budo*). More Westernized people also use the Japanized *wainu* (wie-nuu).

What kind of wine is this?
Kono budoshu wa donna shurui desu ka?
(Koe-no buu-doe-shuu wah doan-nah shuu-rue-e dess kah?)

Wink—*Mekubase* (May-kuu-bah-say).

Hey! That girl winked at me!
Hora! Ano onna-no-ko ga boku ni mekubase wo shimashita!
(Hoe-rah! Ah-no own-nah-no-koe gah boe-kuu nee may-kuu-bah-say oh she-mahssh-tah).

Wise guy, smart alec—*Namaiki na otoko* (Nah-my-kee nah oh-toe-koe).

He is a smart alec.
Anohito wa namaiki na otoko desu.
(Ah-no-ssh-toe wah nah-my-kee nah oh-toe-koe dess.)

"Wolf"—*Ero otoko* (Eh-roe oh-toe-koe).
Also, *sukebe* (sue-kay-bay) and *sukebe komashi* (sue-kay-bay koe-mah-she), which more or less means "playboy."

Woman—*Onna* (Own-nah).
This is the generic term for woman. The specific word is *onna-no-hito* (own-nah-no-ssh-toe), or *onna-no-kata* (own-nah-no-kah-tah), which is a politer form. **Female sex**—*Jo sei* (Joe say-e).

It appears that some Japanese women have a weakness for foreign men.
Aru Nihonjin no onna wa gaijin no otoko ni yowai so desu.
(Ah-rue Nee-hoan-jeen no own-nah wah guy-jeen no oh-toe-koe nee yoe-wah-ee soh dess)

A woman who has the last word—*Kuchi no heranai onna* (Kuu-chee no hay-rah-nie own-nah).
Or, literally, a "woman whose mouth does not run down."

Women's Lib—*Uman Ribu* (Uu-mahn Ree-buu).
Women's liberation groups are active in Japan, but do not appear as strident as some of those in the United States. The workplace remains the last major bastion of male chauvinism in Japan, just as it is in most Western countries.

Woman's sexual peak—*Onna zakari* (Own-nah zah-kah-ree).
A woman's sexual peak (in Japan) is said to be when she is between the ages of 35 and 45, after she has had considerable sexual experience and is fully mature.

Woo (court)—*Kudoku* (Kuu-doe-kuu).
To woo—*Kudoite miru* (Kuu-doy-tay me-rue).

Wooing a woman is very expensive.
Onna wo kudoku ni wa okane ga zuibun kakarimasu.
(Own-nah oh kuu-doe-kuu nee wah oh-kah-nay gah
zuu-ee-boon kah-kah-ree-mahss).

Y

Yoshiwara—*Yoshiwara* (Yoe-she-wah-rah).
This was Japan's most famous pleasure quarter for more than
200 years, until it closed in 1957. The once bustling red-light
district was in the Asakusa area of Tokyo, now noted for its
restaurants, bars, massage parlors and annual festivals. The
Ginza Subway Line (Tokyo's first subway line) begins in
Shibuya on the southwest side of the city and ends in Asakusa
on the northeast side.

You—*Anata* (Ah-nah-tah).
Also, in descending order of politeness: *kimi* (kee-me); *temei*
(tah-may-e). Don't use the latter unless you are looking for
a fight. The plural of you is *anata-tachi* (ah-nah-tah-tah-chee)
or anata-gata (ah-nah-tah-gah-tah), which is more polite.

I'm mad about you.
Anata ni netchu shite imasu.
(Ah-nah-tah nee nate-chuu ssh-tay ee-mahss.)

I'm crazy about you.
Anata ni muchu desu.
(Ah-nah-tah nee muu-chuu dess.)

I can't live without you.
Anata nashi de wa ikite irarenai.
(An-nah-tah nah-she day wah ee-kee-tay ee-rah-ray-nie.)

I fell in love with you at first sight.
Hitome mite aishimashita.
(Shh-toe-may me-tay aye-she-mahssh-tah.)

I just want to be good friends with you.
Anata to wa tomodachi dake de itai
(Ah-nah-tah toe wah toe-moe-dah-chee dah-kay day ee-tie).

Young—*Wakai* (Wah-kie).

You are still too young.
Anata wa mada wakasugimasu.
(Ah-nah-tah wah mah-dah wah-kah-suu-ghee-mahss.)

I wish I had come to Japan when I was younger.
Motto wakai toki ni Nihon ni kite itara yokatta.
(Moat-toe wah-kie toe-kee nee Nee-hoan nee kee-tay
ee-tah-rah yoe-kot-tah.)

Z

Zeal—*Nesshin* (Nay-sheen).

Please put a little more zeal into it.
Mo sukoshi nesshin ni yatte kudasai.
(Moh suu-koe-she nay-sheen nee yaht-tay kuu-dah-sie.)